Psychodynamic Formulation

T0335589

Psychodynamic Formulation

By

Deborah L. Cabaniss

and

Sabrina Cherry

Carolyn J. Douglas

Ruth L. Graver

Anna R. Schwartz

Columbia University, Department of Psychiatry, New York, USA

WILEY-BLACKWELL

A John Wiley & Sons, Ltd., Publication

This edition first published 2013, © 2013 by John Wiley & Sons Ltd.

Wiley-Blackwell is an imprint of John Wiley & Sons, formed by the merger of Wiley's global Scientific, Technical and Medical business with Blackwell Publishing.

Registered office: John Wiley & Sons, Ltd, The Atrium, Southern Gate, Chichester, West Sussex, PO19 8SQ, UK
Editorial offices: 9600 Garsington Road, Oxford, OX4 2DQ, UK
                       The Atrium, Southern Gate, Chichester, West Sussex, PO19 8SQ, UK
                       2121 State Avenue, Ames, Iowa 50014-8300, USA

For details of our global editorial offices, for customer services and for information about how to apply for permission to reuse the copyright material in this book please see our website at www.wiley.com/wiley-blackwell.

Library of Congress Cataloging-in-Publication Data

Psychodynamic formulation / by Deborah L. Cabaniss ... [et al.].
    p. ; cm.
  Includes bibliographical references.
  ISBN 978-1-119-96234-2 (cloth)
  I. Cabaniss, Deborah L.
  [DNLM: 1. Mental Disorders–diagnosis. 2. Mental Disorders–therapy. 3. Patient Care Planning. 4. Psychoanalytic Therapy–methods. WM 141]
  616.89–dc23

                                                                                      2012047255

A catalogue record for this book is available from the British Library.

Wiley also publishes its books in a variety of electronic formats. Some content that appears in print may not be available in electronic books.

Cover image: Nicki Averill Design & Illustration

Cover design by Nicki Averill Design & Illustration

Set in 10/12 Palatino by Laserwords Private Limited, Chennai, India.

1 2013

For our families:

Thomas, William and Daniel

Marc, Rebecca and Ruth

Jon, William and Ben

Michael, Sam and Jacob

Eric, Lena and Maia

This book may be seen as a companion to Psychodynamic Psychotherapy: A clinical manual. For details, see www.wiley.com or scan this QR code:

Contents

Acknowledgments   ix
Introduction   xi

PART ONE   Introduction to the Psychodynamic Formulation   1
1   What is a Psychodynamic Formulation?   3
2   How do We Use Psychodynamic Formulations?   8
3   How do We Construct a Psychodynamic Formulation?   12

PART TWO   DESCRIBE   17
4   Self   23
5   Relationships   32
6   Adapting   41
7   Cognition   52
8   Work and Play   61
    Putting it Together – A Description of Problems and Patterns   69

PART THREE   REVIEW   75
9   What We're Born with – Genetics and Prenatal Development   81
10 The Earliest Years   90
11 Middle Childhood   101
12 Later Childhood, Adolescence, and Adulthood   113
    Putting it Together – A Developmental History   123

PART FOUR   LINK   135

13 Trauma   143

14 Early Cognitive and Emotional Difficulties   152

15 Conflict and Defense   163

16 Relationships with Others   173

17 The Development of the Self   182

18 Attachment   191

Putting it Together–A Psychodynamic Formulation   201

PART FIVE   Psychodynamic Formulations in Clinical Practice   213

19 Psychodynamic Formulations in Acute Care Settings   215

20 Psychodynamic Formulation in Pharmacologic Treatment   222

21 Psychodynamic Formulation in Long-Term Psychodynamic
    Psychotherapy: Revising Over Time   230

22 Sharing Formulations with Our Patients   238

Epilogue   247

Appendix – How to Use *Psychodynamic Formulation*: A Guide for
Educators   249

Recommended Reading   253

Index   259

Acknowledgments

Constructing a psychodynamic formulation is one thing, but trying to teach someone else to construct one is something else entirely. It's like trying to teach someone to tie a shoe. You know how to do it, but what are the steps? How do you put things together? What do you have to know in order to do it? This is what my coauthors and I tried to figure out. The result is our DESCRIBE/REVIEW/LINK method and a curriculum that helps students learn why psychodynamic formulations are important and how to construct them from the bottom up. Along the way, Sabrina Cherry and I wrote formulations and discussed our thought process over countless phone calls; Carolyn Douglas helped to keep us balanced between nature and nurture; Ruth Graver helped to devise a wonderful, dimensional way to describe function; and Anna Schwartz reminded us of the centrality of trauma and the utility of formulations in multiple settings. Both *Psychodynamic Psychotherapy: A Clinical Manual* and *Psychodynamic Formulation* would not be what they are if not for this incredible team of women who are outstanding clinicians, educators, and writers. I am, as ever, grateful for their time, effort, creativity, and friendship.

The *beta* version of this book was road-tested by our terrific Columbia residents, and I thank them for putting up with early drafts riddled with typos. Having the opportunity to teach them day in and day out, year after year, keeps us asking the important questions about education. I owe many thanks to Justin Richardson, who helped me to conceptualize new ways of teaching formulation and with whom I taught for 5 years. David Goldberg, Deborah Katz, and Volney Gay are world-class psychodynamics educators whom I have come to rely on for their wisdom and guidance – each of them carefully read the entire manuscript and gave us invaluable comments that helped us to shape the final product. Sarah Paul offered insightful comments as well. Steven Roose kept me on track to think about function rather than disorders, and Roger MacKinnon made sure that psychodynamic formulation would always be a central part of psychiatric training at Columbia. Joan Marsh, our editor at Wiley, has become a friend and I am grateful for her enthusiasm about our work. Maria Oquendo and Melissa Arbuckle continue to support our teaching at Columbia, without which none of this would be possible.

I'd also like to thank the many students and educators who are using and enjoying *Psychodynamic Psychotherapy: A Clinical Manual*. The overwhelmingly positive response we got to the *Manual* energized us write this companion volume. We are delighted that it has helped to make psychodynamic technique more understandable, and we hope that this book does the same for psychodynamic formulation.

Older and wiser than they were when we wrote the first book, my children William and Daniel are now resigned to the idea that their mom likes writing on nights and weekends. I know that they are proud of me and of the work I'm doing. They will be ready to edit the next book. And, once again, Thomas read every word – sometimes twice – and kept the faith even when I didn't. I couldn't do any of it without him.

Deborah L. Cabaniss
New York
September 2012

Introduction

When we look up at the Rocky Mountains, we see some of the most beautiful scenery on Earth. If asked to describe it, we could wax poetic about the snow capped peaks, alpine meadows, and craggy ravines. That's what they are now – that's what we see. But how did the Rockies get to be the Rockies? How did they form? To figure that out, geologists have used information gathered from the rocks themselves, as well as theories about plate tectonics, to hypothesize that the Rockies arose when two continental plates collided. No one on Earth saw this happen – in fact, no one has ever seen a tectonic plate. However, the evidence is good that forces moving beneath the Earth's surface millions of years ago led to the formation of one of the most beautiful places on the globe. These subterranean forces, in addition to millions of years of rain, snow, ice, and wind, made the Rockies what they are today. This hypothesis helps us understand the history of our planet and predict the way the Earth will continue to change in response to forces working below and above the surface.

When we meet adult patients, we see what they are like now. We hear their speech, observe their behaviors, and listen to their ideas. But how did they come to be the way they are? What forces shaped them? Like geologists, psychodynamic psychotherapists look beyond the surface for answers to these questions. They hypothesize that people are shaped by forces working both beneath and above the surface over time, and they believe that thinking about how that happened is important for understanding a person's past, present, and future. Their hypotheses are their **psychodynamic formulations**, and these formulations are essential to every aspect of the way they treat their patients.

Students and clinicians are often needlessly daunted by the prospect of creating psychodynamic formulations, wondering how they can learn about subterranean forces that even their patients cannot easily access. While it takes time and thought, every clinician can learn to construct psychodynamic formulations using three steps:

1. DESCRIBING the patient's problems and patterns
2. REVIEWING the patient's developmental history
3. LINKING the problems and patterns to the history using organizing ideas about development

This book will teach you each of these three steps using clear language and illustrative examples. **Part One** will introduce you to the psychodynamic formulation and the DESCRIBE/REVIEW/LINK method; **Part Two** will teach you to DESCRIBE problems and patterns; **Part Three** will teach you to REVIEW the developmental history; and **Part Four** will teach you the various ways of LINKING the problems and patterns to the history using different organizing ideas about development. **Part Five** will offer ways to use psychodynamic formulations in various clinical situations and settings. Finally, Parts Two–Four are followed by **Putting it Together** sections that offer full, clinical illustrations of the part of the formulation you've just learned about. Note that all of the clinical examples in the book feature fictional people.

A psychodynamic approach to case formulation is unique in that it considers the way the unconscious mind affects our thoughts, feelings, and behavior. However, as psychodynamic psychotherapists, we are interested in everything that has affected and will affect our patients. This includes both nature and nurture. For this reason, we have intentionally included a considerable amount of information about genetics, temperament, and trauma and the way in which they impact development. It is our firm belief that we should not construct psychodynamic formulations in silos – we cannot hypothesize about the development of our unconscious thoughts and feelings without considering the impact of our endowment and early cognitive and emotional problems on that development. Our hope is that this will encourage you to think broadly about the myriad factors that have affected the way your patients think, feel, and behave.

This book is appropriate for medical students, social work students, psychology students, psychiatry residents, and practicing clinicians. It can be used by individuals who are interested in learning about psychodynamic formulation on their own, as well as by students and teachers in educational settings. Our students learn to DESCRIBE in their earliest years of training, to REVIEW developmental histories slightly later, and to LINK once they have a substantial amount of clinical experience (see Appendix for more specifics). Whether you are an individual learner or an educator, we suggest that using *Psychodynamic Formulation* in this stepwise fashion will help you and/or your students to learn to construct psychodynamic formulations without feeling overwhelmed by the task.

Constructing formulations is not just an interesting exercise – it's an essential part of how we treat our patients. Although this book will teach you to *write* a psychodynamic formulation, our true goal is for you to use what you learn here to constantly *think* about psychodynamic formulations for every patient you see. Without psychodynamic formulations, we can only see the surface – we cannot understand the extraordinary forces that work together to shape the way people think, feel, and behave. It is this understanding that helps us to know what our patients need to learn about themselves, and what they need to develop, in order to live more satisfying, freer lives. So, let's move on to begin learning about *Psychodynamic Formulation*.

PART ONE: Introduction to the Psychodynamic Formulation

1 What is a Psychodynamic Formulation?

Key concepts

A formulation is an explanation or hypothesis.

A case formulation is an hypothesis that helps us to answer questions about the way a patient thinks, feels, and behaves.

A psychodynamic formulation is an hypothesis about the way a person thinks, feels, and behaves, which considers the impact and development of unconscious thoughts and feelings.

A person's development is affected by both hereditary and environmental influences, and thus, both should be included in a psychodynamic formulation.

Psychodynamic formulations do not offer definitive explanations; rather, they are hypotheses that we can change over time.

What is a formulation?

Very nice history. Now can you formulate the case?

All mental health trainees have heard this, but what does it mean? How does one formulate a case? Why is it important?

Formulating means explaining – or better still, hypothesizing. All health care professionals construct **formulations** all the time to understand their patients' problems. In mental health fields, the kinds of problems that we are trying to understand involve the way our patients think, feel, and behave. We often call this kind of formulation a **case formulation**. When we formulate cases, we are not only thinking about *what* people think, feel, and behave but also *why* they do. For example,

---

Psychodynamic Formulation, First Edition. Deborah L. Cabaniss, Sabrina Cherry, Carolyn J. Douglas, Ruth L. Graver, and Anna R. Schwartz.
© 2013 John Wiley & Sons, Ltd. Published 2013 by John Wiley & Sons, Ltd.

Why is she behaving this way?

Why does he think that about himself?

Why is she responding to me like this?

Why is that his way of dealing with stress?

Why is she having difficulty working and enjoying herself?

What is preventing him from living the life he wants to lead?

Different etiologies suggest different treatments; thus, having hypotheses about these questions is vital for recommending and conducting the treatment.

What makes a formulation psychodynamic?

There are many different kinds of case formulations [1–3]. There are cognitive behavioral therapy (CBT) formulations, psychopharmacologic formulations, and family systems formulations – just to name a few. Each type of formulation is based on a different idea about what causes the kinds of problems that bring people to mental health treatment.

One way of thinking about this postulates that these problems are often caused by thoughts and feelings that are out of awareness – that is, that are **unconscious**. This is called a **psychodynamic frame of reference**. Thus, a psychodynamic formulation is an hypothesis about the way a person's unconscious thoughts and feelings may be causing the difficulties that have led him/her to treatment. This is important to understand, as helping people to become aware of their unconscious thoughts and feelings is an important psychodynamic technique.

A developmental process

It's well known that psychodynamically oriented mental health professionals are interested in their patients' childhoods. But why? Well, using psychodynamic technique is about more than just helping people to become aware of their unconscious thoughts and feelings – it's also about understanding how and why those unconscious thoughts and feelings developed. We can use that understanding in many different ways when we treat our patients. Sometimes we share this understanding with our patients to help them see that they are behaving as if earlier conditions still persist:

Example

Mr A's mother, while loving, was extremely undependable. For example, she frequently forgot to pick him up from school. As an adult, Mr A has difficulty believing that his friends and lovers will be consistent in their relationships with him. His therapist is able to help him see that this difficulty may have stemmed from his out-of-awareness fear that people in his adult life will behave as his mother did.

At other times, we use this understanding to help patients develop capacities that were not fully formed during their earlier years:

Example

Ms B, a brilliant student, is unable to think highly of her accomplishments. Raised in foster care, she never received praise for her talents. Understanding this, her therapist is able to help her to believe that her perception of herself is not consonant with her abilities. Over time, she is able to develop new ways of managing her self-esteem.

Finally, we can help support patients' functioning that is impaired by acute or chronic problems:

Example

Mr C presents for therapy because he is having difficulty handling his children during his long divorce. He describes feeling that his parents' divorce, which happened early in his life, had catastrophic effects on his development. His therapist helps him to acknowledge his fear that his divorce will permanently damage his children and to understand the way in which this fear is affecting his parenting. This helps him to relax with his children and to develop alternate strategies for engaging them.

Although their techniques are different, each of these therapists uses an understanding of the patient's development to guide the treatment. Thus, our psychodynamic formulations need to include

1. ideas about how unconscious thoughts and feelings might affect our patients' problems
2. ideas about how those unconscious thoughts and feelings might have developed

That's all well and good, but how can we understand a developmental process that has already occurred? Even with camcorders and scrapbooks, we can't go back in time with people to watch their development unfold. In this way, constructing a psychodynamic formulation is a lot like being a detective trying to solve a mystery – the deed is done and we have to look backward and retrace our steps in order to crack the case. Like the detective, we work retrospectively when we construct a psychodynamic formulation – that is, we first look at our patients' problems and patterns and then scroll back through their personal histories to try to understand their development.

Nature or nurture?

So how *do* our characteristic patterns of thinking, feeling, and behaving develop? John Locke said that each person is born as a blank slate – a *tabula rasa* [4]. E. O. Wilson argued that social behavior is shaped almost entirely by genetics [5]. Nature – nurture – we have to believe that it isn't one OR the other but BOTH. Freud called the nature part "constitutional factors" and the nurture part "accidental factors" [6]. However you think about it, people come into the world with a certain genetic loading and then continue to develop as they interact with their environment. The more we learn about the interrelationship between genes and environment, the clearer it is that our genetics shape our experience and vice versa, so some complex interaction between the two results in our characteristic views of ourselves, the way we relate to other people, and our methods for adapting to stress. Thus, in thinking about how to understand and describe how our patients develop, we have to consider genetic, temperamental, and environmental factors.

More than reporting

A news story gives a report of *what* happened; a psychodynamic formulation offers an hypothesis of *why* things happened. Here are two examples to illustrate the difference:

Reporting

Mr D was born prematurely to a teenage mother who had a postpartum depression. He had severe separation anxiety as a child and spent long periods of time home "sick." As an adult, he is unable to be away from his wife for more than one night.

Formulating

Mr D was born prematurely to a teenage mother who had a postpartum depression. He had severe separation anxiety as a child and spent long periods of time home "sick." It is possible that his mother's depression affected Mr D's ability to develop a secure attachment and that this made it hard for him to think of himself as a separate person. This may have impeded his capacity to separate successfully from his mother. Now, it may be making it difficult for him to be apart from his wife for more than one night.

Although both vignettes tell a "story," only the second attempts to link the history and the problem to make an etiological hypothesis. A psychodynamic formulation is more than a story; it is a narrative that tries to explain how and why people think, feel, and behave the way they do based on their development. In the above example, the sentences "It is possible . . . " and "This may have impeded . . . " suggest causative links between Mr A's problem with separation and his history – links of which he is not aware of and are thus unconscious. *These causative links make this a formulation and not just a history.*

Different kinds of psychodynamic formulations

Psychodynamic formulations can explain one or many aspects of the way a person thinks, feels, or behaves. They can be based on a small amount of information (e.g., the history a clinician obtains during a single encounter in an emergency room) or an enormous amount of information (e.g., everything that a psychoanalyst learns about a patient during the course of an analysis). They can try to explain how someone behaves in a moment of therapy, during a discrete crisis, or over a lifetime. They can be used in any treatment setting, for brief or long-term treatments. If they are responses to questions about how people think, feel, and behave that consider the impact and development of unconscious thoughts and feelings, they are psychodynamic formulations.

Not a static process

It's important to remember that a psychodynamic formulation is just an hypothesis. As above, we can never really know what happened, but, in order to understand our patients better, we try to get an idea of what shaped the way they developed. Earlier in the history of psychoanalysis, the psychodynamic formulation was thought to be a definitive explanation of a person's development. Now we understand that it is better conceptualized as a tool to improve our treatment methods and understanding of our patients.

Hypotheses are generated to be tested and revised. The same is true of psychodynamic formulations. The process of creating a psychodynamic formulation does not end when the clinician generates an hypothesis; rather, it continues for as long as the clinician and patient work together. The formulation represents an ever-changing, ever-growing understanding of the patient and his/her development. We can call this a **working psychodynamic formulation**. Over time, both patient and therapist learn about new patterns and new history. With this, new ways of thinking about development may become useful, and these can help generate new hypotheses. The process of describing patterns, reviewing history, and linking the two using organizing ideas about development is repeated again and again during the course of the treatment, shaping and honing both the therapist's and patient's understanding.

Formulating psychodynamically is ultimately a way of thinking

We think that the best way to learn to formulate psychodynamically is to actually write a psychodynamic formulation. Taking the time to do this, as well as forcing yourself to commit your ideas to paper (or screens!), will help you to consolidate your ideas about a patient and to practice the skills that you will learn in this book. But not all formulations are written. In fact, most are not. We formulate psychodynamically all the time – when we listen to patients, when we think about patients, and when we decide what to say to patients. Ultimately, formulating psychodynamically is a way of thinking that happens constantly in a clinician's mind. Our hope is that you will use the skills that you learn in this book to formulate psychodynamically all the time with all your patients.

Now that we have introduced some basic concepts, let's move on to Chapter 2 to further explore the way we use psychodynamic formulations.

2 How do We Use Psychodynamic Formulations?

> ## Key concepts
>
> The psychodynamic formulation is our map – it guides every aspect of the treatment.
> Having a working psychodynamic formulation enables us to
>
> - make treatment recommendations and set goals
> - understand what patients need developmentally
> - develop therapeutic strategies and predict the way patients will react in treatment (transference)
> - construct meaningful interventions
> - help our patients to create cohesive life narratives
>
> Sometimes we share our psychodynamic formulations with our patients, and sometimes we use them privately to help shape our therapeutic strategies and interventions.

Formulation is our map

Having a working psychodynamic formulation means having a continuously evolving idea about the unconscious thoughts and feelings that affect our patients' ways of thinking, feeling, and behaving. But how do we learn about a part of the mind that is out of awareness? We **listen** carefully to what our patients say so that we can pick up clues that might guide us toward unconscious material, we **reflect** on what our patients say, and we **intervene** in ways that help them to learn more about their minds [7]. As we listen, we do not necessarily know where we're going – in psychodynamic psychotherapy, we follow the patient's lead. But the fact that we follow the patient's lead does not mean that we work without a map. That map is our psychodynamic formulation. When we have a sense of our patients' primary problems and patterns, their developmental histories, and how and why they developed as they did, we listen to them with this in mind.

Psychodynamic Formulation, First Edition. Deborah L. Cabaniss, Sabrina Cherry, Carolyn J. Douglas, Ruth L. Graver, and Anna R. Schwartz.
© 2013 John Wiley & Sons, Ltd. Published 2013 by John Wiley & Sons, Ltd.

Using a psychodynamic formulation in treatment

To further explore this, let's consider the example of Ms A. She is a 43-year-old woman who has come for treatment with Dr Z because she is worried that her husband will leave her. She explains that her husband is a "genius" and that she cannot understand why he wants to remain married to someone who just stays home and takes care of the children. She says,

> I've become one of those boring housewives. The only thing I can talk about is the soccer schedule.

Making a treatment recommendation and setting goals

As Dr Z conducts the evaluation, she learns that Ms A is unable to say anything good about herself. Dr Z also recognizes that Ms A's self-effacement seems incongruous given her apparent abilities – she was a gifted painter who gave up her career when she married. Dr Z begins to wonder about why Ms A has this view of herself. As Dr Z takes the developmental history, she learns that Ms A's mother was a world-famous scientist who was critical of her daughter's complete lack of interest in science, preferring Ms A's brother who became a physicist. Dr Z constructs an early **psychodynamic formulation** (hypothesis) that Ms A has unconscious, maladaptive ways of perceiving herself and regulating her self-esteem and that these unconscious self-perceptions and conflicts might have developed as a result of Ms A's problematic relationship with her mother. Although Dr Z knows that she has much more to learn about Ms A, she uses her preliminary formulation to make a **treatment recommendation** and to work with Ms A to **set early goals**, saying:

> It is clear to me that you are worried about your relationship with your husband. However, it also seems that you are overly tough on yourself and that you do not allow yourself to do things that interest you. These difficulties could be related to longstanding feelings you have about yourself that may date back to your early relationship with your mother. Exploring these feelings in a psychodynamic psychotherapy may help us to understand why you are so unhappy in your current situation and help you to improve both your relationship and your feelings about yourself.

Forming a therapeutic strategy

Ms A agrees and she and Dr Z begin a twice-a-week psychodynamic psychotherapy. Dr Z uses her hypothesis that Ms A was not able to develop an adequate sense of self to understand that M has a **developmental need** to improve her self-perception and her capacity for self-esteem regulation. This forms the basis for Dr Z's **therapeutic strategy**; she will listen to everything that Ms A says, paying close attention to material that might relate to Ms A's difficulties with her sense of self.

Conducting the treatment

For example, one year into the treatment, Ms A says to Dr Z,

> You must be tired of me just talking about my problems day after day. You probably have other patients who need your help more than I do.

Dr Z uses her formulation to help Ms A notice her problematic self-perception, saying,

> I think that you presume that I, like your mother, will be disappointed in you and will be more interested in others.

Creating a life narrative

Over time, Ms A begins to believe that Dr Z is, in fact, truly interested in her. Through her conversations with Dr Z, she realizes that she had a distorted expectation that Dr Z, like her mother, would find her dull and lacking. Together, they use this formulation **to create a life narrative** for Ms A, which helps her to make sense of how she developed this maladaptive unconscious fantasy. In Ms A's words,

> I never realized how hurt I was that my mother wasn't as interested in me as she was in my brother. I also never understood the toll that this took on the way I thought about myself. I'm now seeing that my husband isn't uninterested in me – I just presume that everyone is.

As the treatment unfolds, Dr Z deepens and alters her formulation, but she continues to use it to help her to set goals, develop her therapeutic strategy, listen to the patient, construct interventions, and foster Ms A's understanding of her life. It will remain key to every part of the treatment, from beginning to end.

Do we share our formulations with our patients?

Sometimes we share our psychodynamic formulations with our patients, and sometimes we use them privately to shape our therapeutic strategies and interventions. As we'll discuss further in Chapter 22, we make decisions about this based on what we think is most clinically helpful for the patient in that moment. When patients are self-reflective and able to think about the impact and development of their unconscious thoughts and feelings, it can be helpful to share our formulations:

Example

Ms B is a 30-year-old woman who comes to therapy with Mr Y because she is unsure about her upcoming wedding. She says that although she loves her fiancé, she is worried that she will end up being as unhappy a wife as her mother was. In therapy, Ms B and her therapist evolve the hypothesis that Ms B has an unconscious conflict – although she loves her fiancé and wants to spend her life with him, she feels guilty about having the kind of marriage her mother never had. Understanding this allows her to go ahead with her wedding and to feel better about her relationship.

When patients are less self-reflective, it may be more useful to use our formulations privately:

Example

Ms C is a 58-year-old woman whose husband of 25 years died 6 months ago. She comes to the clinic for help with disorganization, explaining to Dr X that she is having trouble doing things like paying bills and balancing her checkbook. After determining that Ms C does not have symptoms of anxiety, depression, or cognitive impairment, Dr X asks Ms C whether her husband had taken care of the household finances. Ms C acknowledges that he had, but says that she doesn't think that her current problems have anything to do with her husband's death: "I've always been independent, so I'll be fine alone." Dr X hypothesizes that Ms C's inability to take over her husband's tasks is related to feelings about having lost her husband, but thinks that Ms C is not ready to talk about this and that she is highly invested in feeling independent. Therefore, Dr X uses her formulation privately to help Ms C develop strategies for doing one task at a time. This helps Ms C to feel more able to approach these tasks and to feel more independent, although she remains unable to discuss how much she misses her husband.

While both Mr Y and Dr X developed psychodynamic formulations about their patients, Mr Y shared his formulation with Ms B, while Dr X used her formulation without explicitly sharing it. But how did these therapists construct their formulations? We will begin to explore that in Chapter 3.

3 How do We Construct a Psychodynamic Formulation?

Key concepts

When we construct psychodynamic formulations, we

DESCRIBE the patient's primary problems and patterns

REVIEW his/her developmental history

LINK the problems and patterns to the history using organizing ideas about development

---

How do we develop hypotheses to explain things we observe? It could be anything – a cultural trend, the relationship between two people, or a natural phenomenon. For example, let's say that people have a sense that there was less snowfall than usual in their town, and they want to know whether this will be a trend. First, they need to define the phenomenon by using careful observation and measurement. Then, they have to research the history of snowfall in the area. Once they've done this, they can use meteorological theories – for example, theories about global warming – to help them link their observations and the history to form an hypothesis about what's happening and what might happen in the future. They can then explain their hypotheses to others in a cogent way.

The three basic steps to create a psychodynamic formulation

We follow the same steps when we construct psychodynamic formulations to help us understand how and why people develop their characteristic patterns of thinking, feeling, and behaving. This process involves three basic steps. We

DESCRIBE the primary problems and patterns

REVIEW the developmental history

LINK the problems and patterns to the history using organizing ideas about development

---

Psychodynamic Formulation, First Edition. Deborah L. Cabaniss, Sabrina Cherry, Carolyn J. Douglas, Ruth L. Graver, and Anna R. Schwartz.
© 2013 John Wiley & Sons, Ltd. Published 2013 by John Wiley & Sons, Ltd.

Taken together, these three steps comprise the formulation. Each step is crucial to the process and is discussed at length in Parts Two–Four; we briefly outline them here by way of introduction.

DESCRIBE the primary patterns and problems

Before we think about *why* people developed their primary problems and patterns, we have to be able to describe *what* they are. Here, we're not just talking about the chief complaint, but about the issues that underlie the person's predominant ways of thinking, feeling, and behaving. We can divide these into five basic areas of function:

- self
- relationships
- adapting
- cognition
- work and play

It is important to describe each of these areas in order to understand the way a person functions. To do this, we learn from what the patient *tells* us as well as from what the patient *shows* us. For example, a patient may say that he/she gets along well with others but then argue with the therapist throughout the evaluation. We have to use both sources of information when we describe his/her relationships with others. It's also essential to have more than just a surface description of each of these functions in order to really understand our patients. We will address all these areas and how to describe them in Part Two.

REVIEW the developmental history

When patients come to see us, we "take a history" to understand the events that led up to the presenting problem. But to construct a psychodynamic formulation, we need to do much more than that. Our goal is to learn everything we can about our patients in order to begin to make links between their histories and the development of their primary problems and patterns. To do this, we have to take a **developmental history**. This kind of history begins before birth, with the patient's family of origin, prenatal development, and genetic endowment; it includes every aspect of the first years of life, including attachment, early relationships with caregivers, and trauma, and it continues through later childhood, adolescence, and adulthood, until the present moment. Since we don't know why people develop their typical patterns, we have to consider everything – we're interested in heredity and environmental factors and the relationship between the two. We want to understand periods of development that went well, as well as periods that were problematic – we need all the information we can get to try to hypothesize causative links between the history and the development of the patient's primary characteristics. Reviewing the developmental history is the subject of Part Three.

LINK the problems and patterns to the history using organizing ideas about development

The final step in constructing a psychodynamic formulation is linking the problems and patterns to the developmental history to form a longitudinal narrative that offers hypotheses about how and why the patient developed his/her ways of thinking, feeling, and behaving. In doing this, we can be helped by **organizing ideas about development**. These organizing ideas offer us different ways of conceptualizing and understanding our patients' developmental experiences. They help us to take the information that we have learned from the history and think about how it could have led to the problems and patterns we see in our patients. Different ideas may be more helpful in understanding different problems and patterns. The organizing ideas that we discuss in Part Four address the impact of the following on development:

- trauma
- early cognitive and emotional difficulties
- conflict and defense
- relationships with others
- the development of the self
- attachment

So let's begin constructing psychodynamic formulations with Part Two – DESCRIBING function.

Part One References

1. Eels TD (ed). *Handbook of Psychotherapy Case Formulation*. Guilford Press: New York, 2007.
2. Campbell WH, Rohrbaugh RM. *The Biopsychosocial Formulation Manual*. Routledge: New York, 2006.
3. Wright JH, Basco MR, Thase ME. *Learning Cognitive-Behavior Therapy*. American Psychiatric Publishing, Inc.: Washington, DC, 2006.
4. Locke J. *An Essay Concerning Human Understanding*. Oxford University Press: Oxford, 1975.
5. Wilson EO. *Sociobiology: The New Synthesis 25th Anniversary Edition*. Harvard University Press: Cambridge, MA, 2000.
6. Freud S. Analysis Terminable and Interminable. In: Strachey, J (ed). *The Standard Edition of the Complete Psychological Works of Sigmund Freud, (1937-1939), Volume XXIII*. Hogarth Press: London, 1937: 209–254.
7. Cabaniss DL, Cherry S, Douglas, CJ, Schwartz, AR. *Psychodynamic Psychotherapy*. Wiley: Oxford, 2011.

PART TWO: DESCRIBE

Introduction

Key concepts

Psychodynamic formulations help us to explain how and why people function the way they do.

Before we try to explain someone's function, we have to be able to DESCRIBE it.

We can do this by describing

- **The Problem** – what brings the patient to treatment now
- **The Person** – the patient's characteristic patterns of thinking, feeling, and behaving

We can divide these into patterns related to

- self
- relationships
- adapting
- cognition
- work and play

We need to describe aspects of function about which the person is aware (conscious) as well as those about which the person is not aware (unconscious).

For each pattern, it is important to think about areas of strength as well as areas of difficulty.

When we think about how something **functions**, we consider whether it does what it was designed to do. A refrigerator is designed to keep food at a low temperature, so if the milk is cold, it is functioning well and if the milk is warm, it is functioning poorly. A car is designed to transport people from place to place, so if it reliably allows us to get around, it is functioning well and if it is always in the shop, it is functioning poorly. Things that are designed to have multiple functions can sometimes work well in one area but not in another. For example, if a desk chair that is meant to be both comfortable and stylish creates a sleek look in an office but leaves workers with backaches, it is fulfilling one function but not the other.

While it's easy to know the intended function of a refrigerator or a car, it's much harder to know what a person is supposed to be able to do. For example, should all people work? Get married? Have children? Belong to a religious organization? Be altruistic? Although some people might believe that all people should be able to do one or all of these things, as mental health professionals it is not our job to make those kinds of judgments. On the contrary, we know that there are as many ways to live as there are people on Earth. However, when people **suffer**, we know that their functioning is faltering in some way.

Before explaining, first describe!

People function by thinking, feeling, and behaving. We construct formulations to try to explain how and why they function the way they do. But we have to be able to describe their function before we can explain it. We can do this by describing both the **Problem** and the **Person**.

Describing the Problem

The **Problem** is what is giving the person the most difficulty *right now*. It is generally, but not always, the reason that he/she gives for consulting a mental health professional. Sometimes we agree with patients about the primary problem and sometimes we don't, but either way we have to acknowledge and address their concerns. Here are a few examples of problems that bring people to psychotherapy:

> *Mr A presented to the clinic for help with understanding his teenage daughter.*
>
> *Ms B consulted a therapist because she is unsure about whether she wants a divorce.*
>
> *Ms C made an appointment because she feels increasingly anxious at work.*
>
> *Mr D was sent for a consultation by his internist because he can't get back on his feet after being fired.*
>
> *Ms E sought therapy because she can't figure out why she's not in a relationship.*

Of course, many patients do not have only one problem. They might have depression and ongoing difficulty with a spouse, or they might drink too much alcohol or have an ailing parent. Nevertheless, it is important to develop the skill to identify and describe what is troubling the person the most right now so that we can try to explain the development of this problem in the psychodynamic formulation. Challenge yourself to answer the question, "Why did this person come to see me *now*?" and you are likely to identify the primary problem.

It is important to get all the details – whether the problem is an interpersonal difficulty or symptoms of a mood or anxiety disorder. When we think psychodynamically, we are also interested in carefully diagnosing our patients' cognitive and emotional difficulties. Understanding that a patient has a major depression, an eating disorder, or substance abuse is central to the way we recommend and conduct treatment. However, constructing psychodynamic formulations requires us to learn more about our patients than we can learn from the current problem alone.

Describing the Person

The **Problem** is what is giving the patient the most difficulty right now. But in order to fully understand the way someone functions, we have to be able to describe the way he/she generally thinks, feels, and behaves. We can call this describing the **Person**. To consider the differences between the **Problem** and the **Person**, consider Ms F and Ms G. Although they have the same problem, they are experiencing it very differently:

> *Ms F is a 35-year-old woman with two children, who has just been left by her husband of 10 years. Fearful, with few friends, Ms F feels desperate and alone. She calls her husband daily, begging him to come home and threatening to hurt herself if he does not. She feels utterly unlovable and is convinced that she can never have another relationship. She is neglecting herself, her children, and her home.*

> *Ms G is a 35-year-old woman with two children, who has just been left by her husband of 10 years. Although she is shocked and upset, she has rallied her friends and family and has been able to retain a good sense of herself. She is focusing on her children and is trying to maintain a stable home so that their lives will be minimally disrupted. Although not ready to date, she is optimistic that she could have another relationship in the future.*

While both Ms F and Ms G have just been left by their husbands, they have reacted to this situation in different ways. This is because Ms F and Ms G functioned very differently before the problem arose. This functioning is what we refer to as the **Person**; thus, we have to know who the person is as well as the problem that he/she has.

Describing patterns helps one to describe the Person

We can describe the **Person** by describing a patient's characteristic ways of thinking, feeling, and behaving. We can call these his/her characteristic **patterns**. By the time they are adults, people develop characteristic patterns in several aspects of their lives. Throughout the ages, observers of human behavior have used different methods to describe people's characteristic ways of functioning. Some of these methods have attempted to put people into **categories**, based on certain shared features. Hippocrates categorized people according to their balance of four essential bodily fluids [1], Freud grouped people according to their fixations along a psychosexual developmental pathway [2], and the DSM (Diagnostic and Statistical Manual of Mental Disorders) categorizes people using lists of shared characteristics [3]. However, more and more researchers in this area find that describing people's characteristic patterns of thinking and behaving according to certain **dimensions** provides the best way to understand them [4, 5]. In this book, we take a dimensional approach, using five basic areas of function:

- self
- relationships
- adapting
- cognition
- work and play

We describe each area in more depth using a series of **variables**. Learning about and being able to describe every patient's functioning in each of these areas is essential to learning about him/her as a person. How and why a person develops one pattern vs. another is an important aspect of what we want to explain in our psychodynamic formulation. We describe each of these areas, including the basics of the area, common patterns in that area, and ways to assess the area, in Chapters 4–8.

Strengths and difficulties

People are complex, and even within one area of function, they may have strengths and difficulties. Some other people function very well in one area but have more difficulty in another. Consider the following examples:

> Mr H is a 35-year-old heterosexual man who has never had a long-term romantic relationship with a woman. However, he has many close friends, both men and women, with whom he socializes and confides.

> Ms I is a 55-year-old CEO of a major company. She is an excellent manager and a brilliant businesswoman; however, she is extremely anxious in social situations and becomes uncomfortable when she has unstructured time on the weekends.

In terms of his relationship patterns, Mr H's capacity to have close friendships is a strength, while he has difficulty with romantic partners. In the case of Ms I, her outstanding work function is a clear strength, while her relationships and leisure function give her much more difficulty. Like most people, these people are **mosaics**, with good function in one area and more difficulty in another.

Sometimes, as mental health professionals, we focus exclusively on problems and neglect areas of strength and resilience. However, we need to rely on our patients' strengths to help them build new, healthier ways of functioning. Describing our patients' strengths and difficulties allows us to hypothesize about both in our psychodynamic formulations.

Conscious and unconscious patterns

People are aware of some, but not all, of the ways in which they think, feel, and behave. Consider Ms J and Ms K:

> Ms J is a 35-year-old woman who presents for therapy saying, "I have so much trouble feeling good about myself. I've always been like that, ever since I was a child. It's something I'd like to work on."
>
> Ms K is a 35-year-old woman who presents for therapy saying, "My husband said that it was either therapy or divorce. He says that I don't listen to him. Why should I? He drones on all the time about his work – accounting – what could be more boring? By the way, you need a new receptionist. She mispronounced my name twice – not too bright."

Ms J is conscious that she has difficulties with self-esteem, even if she's not aware of why she does. Conversely, we can hypothesize that Ms K has unconscious difficulties with self-esteem, which are suggested by her tendency to belittle others in order to feel good about herself. When we think psychodynamically, we are interested in both conscious and unconscious patterns.

Looking ahead

Each area of function is important, and allowing ourselves to learn about all of them is essential to describe our patients. Let's move on, then, to Chapter 4 and patterns related to the self.

4 Self

Key concepts

By the time they are adults, people develop characteristic patterns of experiencing themselves. We can describe these patterns using the following variables:

- self-perception, including
  - identity
  - fantasies about the self
- self-esteem, including
  - vulnerability to self-esteem threats
  - internal response to self-esteem threats
  - use of others to regulate self-esteem

Failed exams, breakups, job loss, medical illness – life is full of experiences that threaten our sense of who we are and our ability to feel good about ourselves. Why do some people cope with these situations without loss of self-esteem, while others are devastated? In order to begin to make hypotheses about this, we need to be able to describe the characteristic ways a person experiences his or her **self** [6].

Defining the area: self

Everything we do in life, from having relationships with others to choosing what we do for work and play, relates to how we think about ourselves – that is, to our **self-experience**. Having a realistic idea of what we can do and what we like to do helps us to choose relationships and activities that bring us satisfaction and pleasure and to maintain good feelings about ourselves even in the face of adversity. Thus, our self-experience is central to the way we function.

Psychodynamic Formulation, First Edition. Deborah L. Cabaniss, Sabrina Cherry, Carolyn J. Douglas, Ruth L. Graver, and Anna R. Schwartz.
© 2013 John Wiley & Sons, Ltd. Published 2013 by John Wiley & Sons, Ltd.

Variables for describing patterns related to the self

We can describe a person's self-experience using two major variables:

- self-perception
- self-esteem regulation

Self-perception

When we write "identifying information" about people in a psychological or medical history, we usually start with a sentence that outlines certain things about them, such as their age, gender, employment, and relationship status. When we think about people's self-perception in a psychodynamic formulation, however, we have to consider not only their demographics but also their conscious and unconscious thoughts and feelings about themselves. This includes their sense of **identity** and their **fantasies about themselves**.

Identity

Our sense of **identity** is our sense of who we are [7]. This includes our ability to know our likes and dislikes as well as our talents and limitations. As we'll explore further in Chapter 12, our sense of identity grows through life, particularly during adolescence. Adults with a secure sense of identity use it to make choices about everything, from relationships to career options. Adults with a less secure sense of identity often have difficulty making choices and may have a more erratic life trajectory. Consider the following examples:

> *Mr A is a 27-year-old gay man who is in a master's program in engineering. In college, he did well as a chemistry major and then took an inspiring engineering class; he is now hoping to combine his interests by specializing in chemical engineering. He says, "I'm good at math and science, but not so great at writing, so even though I once thought I wanted to write novels I think that's not in the cards – and I really enjoy what I'm doing." He is in a long-term relationship and hopes one day to have children with his partner.*

> *Mr B is a 27-year-old heterosexual man who is working as a waiter and living with college friends. He says, "I should figure out something else to do but I don't know what that would be. I studied biology in college because my parents told me I should but I kind of hated it. Maybe I'll try writing a novel . . . seems like a good way to make some money but I don't know if I'm much of a writer." Mr B has had brief, intense relationships with women and says, "I don't think I've ever dated someone I liked all that much."*

Although they are at similar points in their lives, Mr A has a much more consolidated sense of identity than Mr B. Mr A is comfortable with his likes and dislikes, both in work and in his relationships, and he has a good sense of his talents and limitations. On the contrary, Mr B is unsure of what he enjoys and is not able to identify his strengths and difficulties.

Fantasies about the self

A student imagines being praised by a teacher for an assignment well done, a teenage boy imagines going on a date with a girl he likes, a scientist imagines winning a Nobel Prize, a retired man imagines being a beloved grandfather – at all stages of life, **fantasies about the self** provide us with comfort, goals, and escapes [8, 9]. They also help us to move forward, strive, and achieve. People whose fantasies about themselves are accurately attuned to their talents and limitations are more likely to feel good about themselves than those who cling to personal goals that are not consonant with their abilities [10].

People have both conscious and unconscious fantasies about themselves. While they may be able to tell us their conscious fantasies, we have to learn about their unconscious fantasies in other ways – for example, by listening to their dreams and by noticing their behaviors.

Example

Ms C, a 44-year-old woman who has never been married, presents for therapy with symptoms of depression. She says that she first felt sad a few weeks after her younger sister's wedding. When the therapist asks whether she might feel bad that her sister married first, Ms C says, "Not at all. I've never wanted to get married. I prefer to be a bridesmaid than a bride. I don't know why I became upset after the wedding – my toast was the highlight of the evening."

Although Ms C consciously experiences herself as the perennial bridesmaid, her depression after her sister's wedding, as well as what sounds like a wish to have "stolen the show," suggests that she may have unconscious fantasies about taking center stage as a bride herself.

Self-esteem regulation

Esteem is respect or admiration, so self-esteem is the respect or admiration we have for ourselves. Most of us begin life excited by our abilities – think of the joy on babies' faces when they say their first words or take their first steps. But maintaining self-esteem in the face of everything that happens to us during life can sometimes feel like a never-ending obstacle course. The ability to pick oneself up after disappointments or slights is called **self-esteem regulation** and is an important part of how people function in the world [11, 12].

Anything that imperils a person's good feelings about himself/herself is a **self-esteem threat** (also called a **narcissistic injury**) [13]. Since people vary in the way they perceive and respond to self-esteem threats, we can use the following variables to describe individual patterns of self-esteem regulation:

- vulnerability to self-esteem threats
- internal response to self-esteem threats
- use of others to help regulate self-esteem

Vulnerability to self-esteem threats

Some people can maintain their positive self-regard in the face of massive emotional injuries, such as severe medical illness or job loss, while others crumble if someone looks at them the wrong way on the street. People who are very vulnerable to self-esteem threats are sometimes said to have **fragile self-esteem**. Consider the difference between Mr D and Ms E:

Mr D, a 50-year-old man with a wife, two children, and a large mortgage, was laid off after 20 years at the same job. He was quite surprised and shaken by the experience. After many late-night discussions with his wife, they decided that for the next year she would return to nursing, which she had done prior to having children, and he would assume the primary child care role while looking for a new job. Although he initially felt a bit sheepish on the playground with the "moms," he enjoyed being closer to his children's lives, used the time to do more physical exercise, and ultimately found a job that was more in line with his interests. In his journal, he wrote that the year had helped him to become a better person.

Ms E, a 26-year-old single woman, began to have some mild acne on her face. As a result, she became distraught, avoided social situations, and worried constantly that she would never have a long-term relationship.

For the family breadwinner, the loss of a job is enough to make anyone lose some self-regard. Yet, despite some anxiety, Mr D is able to right himself and to create a situation in which he has minimal loss of self-esteem. In contrast, Ms E's sense of self completely crumbles when she has a relatively minor cosmetic problem. We would say that Ms E is more vulnerable to self-esteem threats than Mr D. Sometimes people have particular types of self-esteem threats to which they are especially vulnerable. For example, a person might be able to handle critiques from people at work but be very sensitive to criticism from a parent.

Self-esteem vulnerability is often apparent in the way someone reacts to being compared with others. Some people have no difficulty maintaining good feelings about themselves when they lack something that others have, while others find this intolerable. When people are so unable to tolerate this situation that they need to destroy what others have, we say that they are **envious**; if they just want to be on par with others, we say that they are **jealous** [14].

Examples

Walking into a party, Ms F sees an acquaintance wearing a dress that she knows is more expensive than she could afford. In a loud voice, Ms F says, "Some people wear the most garish outfits. It's so inappropriate." She feels good when she sees the acquaintance blush and walk out of the room.

At the same party, Ms G sees a woman wearing a scarf in a fashion that she admires. She momentarily feels that her own outfit looks dated. She makes a mental note to try to buy the same scarf so that she can wear it in that way. The next day, she runs out to buy it.

Ms F is envious; she needs to destroy the other woman's enjoyment of having the dress. On the contrary, Ms G is jealous; as long as she has the new scarf, she does not need to destroy the other woman's experience of having it as well.

Internal response to self-esteem threats

When people experience a threat to their sense of self, they respond in a way that helps them to buoy their self-esteem. This entire process may occur unconsciously. The mechanisms they use to buoy their good feelings about themselves begin to develop in childhood and coalesce into fairly stable patterns by adulthood. More adaptive patterns restore positive feelings flexibly while maintaining other functions, such as relationships with others. Less adaptive patterns are more brittle and often jeopardize other functions and relationships [15].

Less adaptive internal responses

Less adaptive internal responses to self-esteem threats include inflating or deflating one's sense of self. **Grandiosity** is a massive and unwarranted overconfidence that protects people from the pain of facing their limitations. People who rely on grandiosity are often described as **narcissistic** [16]. They tend to externalize their failures, become enraged and demanding, and belittle others. They are unaware that although this allows them to preserve their self-esteem, it is often at the expense of their relationships with others. Consider Ms H:

> Ms H is a 32-year-old woman who is supported by her parents and who would like to be a writer. She says that she has heard you can make a lot of money writing screenplays and that she has a great idea for one she is planning to write. Although she has never had anything published, she says that she's "more talented than most of the hacks out there." In addition, she says that she has the name of a VIP in the TV industry and she is sure it will "just take one phone call."

In contrast, deflating one's sense of self leads to **self-deprecation** and **masochism** [17]. Unable to think of redeeming qualities about themselves, people who respond in this way often self-sabotage and deny their own needs:

> Ms I is a 32-year-old woman who is supported by her parents and who would like to be a writer. She says that she's sure that she'll never succeed in writing because she really has no talent. She downplays the fact that she has already had several pieces published, saying, "they were all in minor magazines." She is currently taking a writing course at the extension division of a local community college. At the end of her first assignment, her teacher wrote, "Really good! Looking forward to your next draft," which Ms H interpreted to mean that the piece was terrible.

In the face of failure, both of these function poorly, often leading to depression and even the risk of suicide.

More adaptive internal responses

People with more adaptive responses may react to self-esteem threats by **becoming more or less competitive**. Although these responses may have less impact on the person's global ability to function, they may still cause difficulties and distress. Consider these examples:

> Growing up with an older sister who was a star athlete on three varsity teams, Ms J has always been a very competitive tennis player. Although she has become good, many people don't like to play with her because of her abrasive manner and her insistence on keeping score during casual games.

Mr K owns a catering company that is doing very well. After becoming very anxious while competing with colleagues for "important events," he now often "forgets" to get his bid in on time for big jobs. He says, "I prefer to stay small," although he sometimes tells his wife that he wishes that he could make more money.

Ms J deals with feelings of insecurity by becoming more competitive, while Mr K deals with similar feelings by staying on the sidelines.

The most adaptive responses to self-esteem threats tend to be flexible and to utilize the most adaptive defenses (see Chapter 6). Humor, sublimation, and altruism help people to restore good feelings about themselves without sacrificing other functions or relationships.

Example

Mr L was unable to pursue his dream of going to law school because he had to take care of his dying mother. He took over the family business and made a comfortable living. He was able to pay for his brother, M, to go to law school, and he is proud of M despite some feelings of regret about his own failed plans. When M complains about how difficult his courses are, Mr L laughs and puts his arm around him, saying, "Don't worry, you'll do fine on your exams. And you'll have to help me out in my old age!"

Altruism and humor help Mr L to deal with a profound disappointment that could have derailed his good feelings about himself.

Use of others to help regulate self-esteem

We all desire admiration from the people we love. Nothing feels as good as hearing "great work!" for a job well done. When given in appropriate amounts, admiration is central to the development of self-esteem (see Chapter 17). Some people, however, require constant attention, praise, and validation from others to manage their self-esteem. They fish for compliments, repeatedly ask for validation, and make themselves the center of attention – often to such a degree that they deplete family and friends with their constant demands. These people require the input of others in order to regulate their self-esteem. They may even act as if other people exist solely to boost their self-esteem, indicating a lack of **empathy** (see Chapter 5) [18].

Examples

When Ms N's therapist told her that she was going to be out for 3 months of maternity leave, Ms N cried and said, "I can't believe that you're going to be out then. That's right when I'm going to have my annual review – it will be the hardest time of the year for me!"

After work, Mr O launches directly into talking to his wife about his day and asking her whether she thinks that he made good decisions before even kissing her hello.

Ms N displays a striking lack of empathy in thinking only of the way her therapist helps her to maintain her self-esteem. Similarly, Mr O sees his wife as existing only to validate his own experiences.

People with more adaptive self-esteem regulation strategies are able to take advice, metabolize it, and make their own decisions. They take pleasure and pride in their accomplishments without relying exclusively on others for praise.

Example

On her way home from work, Ms P smiled to herself as she recalled what a good job she had done on her presentation. When she arrived home, she made dinner and helped her children with their homework. Although she didn't discuss her day with anyone, she went to bed with a good feeling.

Ms P was able to feel good about her work performance without input from anyone else.

Learning about patterns related to the self

Learning about someone's patterns related to the self involves active listening and questioning. The following are some guidelines to help you understand this critical area of functioning:

Learning about self-perception

Sometimes direct questions about identity and fantasies can be helpful. For example:

> *Do you think that you have an accurate sense of your strengths and difficulties? What do others say about that? Do they tend to think that you can do more than you think that you can?*

> *Do you think that you won't be able to do things that you actually can – or is it the other way around?*

> *Would people describe you as someone who knows who he/she is?*

Learning about self-esteem

Learning about self-esteem vulnerability

Asking direct questions about envy, jealousy, and self-esteem vulnerability can make people anxious and defensive. Instead, try asking questions about common situations to learn about this area:

> *How do you feel when you're in a group of people who seem to be wealthier/more accomplished/more highly educated than you are?*

> *Tell me about a time when you didn't get something you really wanted. How did it make you feel?*

> *How do you feel when a friend accomplishes something that you haven't been able to do?*

> *All people have things that make them feel less than good about themselves. What kinds of things make you feel that way?*

Learning about internal responses to self-esteem threats

Listen for stories that have to do with disappointments or failures, and ask questions that will help you to learn about the person's response. For example:

> *Do you tend to feel that others around you are incompetent?*
>
> *Do you generally feel like the smartest/least intelligent person in the room?*
>
> *Do you think that people would tend to describe you as a competitive person?*
>
> *How do you generally go about getting something you want?*

Learning about use of others for self-esteem regulation

> *Do you know when you've done a good job without needing to hear praise from others?*
>
> *Are you able to make decisions without input from others?*

Describing self-experience

Using the variables outlined earlier, here's how we might describe Mr Q's patterns related to the self:

> *In his patterns related to his sense of self, Mr Q has prominent difficulties and some strengths. He has difficulty with **self-perception**, as evidenced by his prediction that he will be promoted to manager despite repeated negative annual reviews. This suggests that he has grandiose **fantasies of the self** that are not consonant with his actual abilities. He has a fairly consolidated **identity** related to his family, as he is proud of being an involved father of two teenage daughters. He has significant difficulty with **self-esteem**. Although Mr Q can tolerate minor **self-esteem threats**, such as being cut off by another driver on the highway, he is extremely vulnerable to more significant threats, such as being criticized by his boss at work. These threats lead him to become irritable and intolerant of others, including his wife and children (**internal response to self-esteem threat**). He frequently **uses others for self-esteem regulation**; for example, at dinner, he will often talk exclusively about himself and his accomplishments. He also tends to have friends who are younger than he is and who look up to him, and he will occasionally flirt with young women in the office whom he is convinced see him as very attractive.*

As we can see from this example, self-experience also has a major impact on relationships, which is the subject of Chapter 5.

Variables for describing the SELF

Self-perception
>   identity
>
>   fantasies about the self

Self-esteem
   vulnerability to self-esteem threats
   internal responses to self-esteem threats
   use of others to regulate self-esteem

Suggested activity

How would you describe Mr A's patterns related to the self?

Mr A is a 43-year-old man who is married and has two children. He has had many different jobs over the years – he drifts from job to job without a real sense of direction. At one point, he decided that he wanted to be an artist and gave up his job, rented a nearby garage, and began painting – despite never having had any art training. He has contempt for people who "settle" for "mainstream" careers, despite the fact that he often envies their lifestyles. "They're working stiffs, but they get everything good in life," he complains. His wife and children have followed him in his meanderings – when they get frustrated, he says that they don't appreciate him.

Comment

Mr A has difficulty with **self-perception** and **self-esteem regulation**. His sense of **identity** is poorly formed, as evidenced by his vague career trajectory. His attempt to become a painter without training or indication of aptitude suggests that his **fantasies about himself** are not consonant with his realistic talents and limitations. He **regulates self-esteem** by becoming grandiose and contemptuous of others, and he is exquisitely **vulnerable to self-esteem threats**. His lack of empathy for the difficulties he is causing his family members suggests that he **uses others to help regulate his self-esteem**.

5 Relationships

Key concepts

The capacity to have relationships is central to the way people function and develop. We can describe a person's relationship patterns according to the following variables:

- trust
- sense of self and other
- security
- intimacy
- mutuality

For most of us, relationships with family, friends, significant others, and colleagues provide us with some of the most rewarding experiences of our lives. Yet, relationships can also be a source of frustration, pain, and confusion. For example, consider a smart but lonely 32-year-old man who is always attracted to unavailable women, or an ambitious middle-aged woman who continuously thwarts her chances for promotion by alienating her bosses. By the time we are adults, we tend to form relationships according to certain patterns which can be more or less adaptive. Being able to describe these patterns is central to understanding how people function [19, 20].

Defining the area: relationships

Relationships are the interactions that we have with people in our lives. There are many different kinds of relationships: the parent–child relationships of early childhood, the peer friendships of later childhood, and the romantic and sexual relationships of adulthood. Relationships can be fleeting or long-term, deep or superficial. Some people have many relationships, while others have few. Most people are capable of having many different types of relationships.

Variables for describing patterns related to relationships

We can describe a person's patterns of relationships with others using the following five variables:

Psychodynamic Formulation, First Edition. Deborah L. Cabaniss, Sabrina Cherry, Carolyn J. Douglas, Ruth L. Graver, and Anna R. Schwartz.
© 2013 John Wiley & Sons, Ltd. Published 2013 by John Wiley & Sons, Ltd.

- trust
- sense of self and other
- security
- intimacy
- mutuality

Trust

The ability to **trust** others is essential for having meaningful, mutually satisfying relationships. This could be a relationship with a family member, a lover, a spouse, or a colleague. Trust allows people to count on one another, to believe that they will be taken care of, and to have confidence in the consistency of their relationships. Lack of trust leads to constant fear of aggression from others, a sense of being neglected, and a perennial feeling of aloneness.

Trust in others develops during the earliest years and depends on both temperament and early relationships with caregivers (see Chapter 10) [21–23]. But before we can think about the origin of a person's capacity to trust, we first have to be able to determine whether or not that trust exists. Let's consider these examples of two 70-year-old men who present for therapy with the chief complaint that they don't know what to do with themselves since retiring:

> Mr A says that his company "tossed him out" after years of good service because, "it's a dog eat dog world out there." Although married, he says that his wife spends most of her time with her family because, "I guess blood is thicker than water." He no longer speaks to most of his friends and acquaintances because, "they all just want money from you in the end." When his therapist suggests that he is depressed and could benefit from medication and therapy, he says, "Yeah, how much did the drug companies pay you to say that?"

> Mr B is a small businessman who just turned over his store to his son. "He'll do a great job," he says, "and I want him to be able to give his family the same good life that I gave my kids, but I still want to feel that I'm doing something useful." He came to therapy at the suggestion of a close friend with whom he has shared his misgivings about retirement. "It's tricky to shift roles – I think that I can do it but I want to talk it through."

Both Mr A and Mr B are facing challenging moments of transition that could be difficult for anyone. Mr A is having more difficulty, however, because he does not trust that others care about him. This has led to a lifelong pattern of vigilance, bitterness, and isolation. On the other hand, Mr B trusts that others care about him and, at age 70, is cushioned by loving relationships. These differences are also clear in the way the two men approach therapy.

Being overly trusting can be problematic, too – the person who trusts everyone or who trusts people he/she shouldn't may also have difficulties with trust. But having at least one or two people who you really trust is vital for adaptive functioning.

Sense of self and other

Being able to think about oneself and others in a three-dimensional way is critical to having healthy relationships [24, 25]. When we say three-dimensional, we mean that the person can think about himself/herself and others as having

- both bad and good qualities
- separate and unique feelings, beliefs, needs, or motivations
- generally consistent feelings about self and others from past to present

Consider the way in which these two people think about their bosses:

Example

Mr C says that his boss, D, is a "jerk" who only cares about his own promotion. He "loved" D when he was recruited, but this shifted when he did not get what he considered to be adequate personal attention. When Mr C's bonus was not what he thought that it should be, he monopolized D's attention, calling and demanding meetings all day, despite the fact that D supervises over 50 people. When D explained that everyone in the department had to take a bonus cut, Mr C vilified D for being weak and considered quitting.

Mr E thinks that his boss, F, is smart and creative but a bit passive. When he didn't get the bonus he thought he deserved, he made an appointment to discuss this with F. F explained that the department had not done as well as anticipated that quarter and that everyone had taken a hit. Mr E was disappointed, and even wondered if perhaps F had not made "enough of a case" for him with the "higher-ups," but also understood the pressure that F was under himself. He generally works well with F and likes his candor and collegiality but is sometimes frustrated by his less aggressive nature.

Both Mr C and Mr E were disappointed and frustrated with their bosses. However, Mr C could see only one side of the story and only one aspect of D, while Mr E could appreciate F's complex nature. Mr C oscillated between "loving" and "hating" D, while Mr E realized that F had multiple sides to his personality – some of which he liked more than others. Mr C's way of thinking about D is called **splitting** [26] – that is, seeing people as all good or all bad (see Chapters 6 and 10). While splitting is normal in small children, it is quite maladaptive if it persists and prevents people like Mr C from being able to think about others three-dimensionally. In addition, it is difficult for Mr C to imagine D as separate from himself – as far as he's concerned, D's whole job is to take care of him. Consequently, it is difficult for him to have an ongoing, meaningful relationship with D, while Mr E, despite his frustration, is able to work with F over time. These issues can also impair a person's ability to think in a more nuanced way about himself/herself, leading to a chronically impoverished or grandiose sense of self (see Chapter 4).

Mr E's ability to think about what might be going on in F's mind also helps him to think about himself and others three-dimensionally. This has been called **mentalization** (see Chapters 6, 10, and 18), which is the ability to think about others as having thoughts and feelings that are distinct from one's own [27, 28].

Security

The word **security** refers to the state of being safe; security in a relationship refers to feeling safe with another person [29, 30]. This means being able to feel that the relationship will persist even if there are

- physical separations
- disagreements
- other negative feelings

In development, this is often called having a **secure attachment** (see Chapters 10 and 18) [31]. People with more secure relationships are generally able to

- tolerate a range of ambivalent feelings about other people
- have a variety of long-lasting relationships
- form relationships more slowly, taking time to get to know others [32]

Consider the following examples:

> Ms G, a 29-year-old graduate student who cannot finish her thesis, recently broke up with her boyfriend after she thought he flirted with her best friend at a party. He denies her charge and says that he has often noticed her flirting with other men. She is angry and refuses to see either her boyfriend or her best friend. She tells you that she met a new guy a week ago and says, "I think I'm in love, he's perfect!" She has moved all her belongings to the new boyfriend's apartment.

> Ms H is a 29-year-old graduate student who is about to finish her thesis. She lives with her boyfriend of 2 years; they've talked about getting married after she settles into her new job in a year or so. Her boyfriend's closest friend is a woman colleague. While Ms F was mildly anxious about this at first, she has now formed a close friendship with the woman. She occasionally jokes about how silly she was to be worried.

Because Ms H is more secure in her relationships than Ms G she is less threatened by the presence of another woman. This allows her to maintain the relationship despite her anxiety.

Intimacy

Intimacy refers to closeness and familiarity. People are intimate with one another if they share things about themselves, such as feelings, experiences, wishes, and disappointments. The degree of intimacy that people generally share with others is an important aspect of their relationship patterns [33]. Depending on the type of relationship, intimacy manifests in different ways. Between lovers, sexuality may be an important way of being intimate; between friends, sharing stories, hopes, and fears might forge intimacy. Without at least some intimacy, relationships are superficial. However, because intimacy involves sharing private thoughts and feelings, it makes many people feel anxious and vulnerable.

Some people tend toward extremes, sharing either too much or too little, while others are better able to modulate their degree of intimacy:

Example

Mr I, a 34-year-old man, meets a woman at a bar and tells her the story of his last three relationships before the second drink.

Mr J, a 34-year-old man, lived with his boyfriend for 3 years before he shared with him that he had a schizophrenic brother.

Both Mr I and Mr J have anxiety about being close to their partners but they handle it in opposite ways; Mr I tells too much too fast, while Mr J is withholding.

Patients often use the word "intimacy" when they talk about having sex, as in, "I was intimate with my girlfriend last night." However, just because two people are having sex does not mean that they are truly intimate. It is important to determine whether people are sharing feelings and private thoughts with their sexual partners before we can say that their relationships are really intimate.

Mutuality

Consider these situations: a friendship in which one person constantly talks about himself/herself while the other listens, a couple who both work full time but one does all the housework, and a baseball-loving father who forces his reluctant son to play little league every year. Each of these situations feels unfair, because it seems as if one person is doing all the giving, while the other does all the taking. The takers have a limited capacity for empathy (see Chapter 4) and thus do not consider the needs of others. Without this, relationships are unbalanced and lack mutuality. The givers may be more empathic, but they also are missing something about what makes a relationship balanced. Relationships are mutual when both people involved are able to give and take [34, 35]. It's a two-way street. Consider Ms K and Ms L:

Ms K is perennially angry with her 16-year-old daughter for spending more time with her friends than with her family. Ms K refuses to let her daughter go to a school dance because there is a family party for a little-known cousin on the same day.

Ms L, a stay-at-home mom, spends every day shuttling her children to and from their many activities. She lacks any time for herself. As soon as they are home, her children run up to their rooms to play video games, while Ms L busies herself with housework. She feels guilty about having occasional thoughts that her children are selfish and spoiled.

While Ms L gives too much and Ms K takes too much, both create relationships that lack mutuality.

Variability in relationship patterns

As with all areas of function, people may have pockets of strength and difficulty. For example, a person may be able to be emotionally intimate with friends but not with romantic partners. Another person might have a very secure relationship with his/her partner but lack sexual intimacy. Finally, people may have strengths in some aspects of their relationships while having difficulty in others. For example, two people who live together and care for each other might have security and mutuality but lack intimacy because they don't tell each other anything private. Clarifying this variability in relationship patterns is essential for understanding this critical area of functioning.

Learning about relationships

Learning about trust

You can ask people about trust in a very straightforward way. During your initial assessment, try asking questions such as

> Is there someone in the world whom you really trust?
>
> Whom do you trust most in your life?
>
> Do you think that person would help you in an emergency?
>
> Do you think that person really cares about you?
>
> Do you generally feel that people will look out for you?
>
> Do you think that I am likely to be able to help you?

Learning about one's sense of self and others

You can start by asking

> Tell me about someone who is important to you. What is he/she like?

If this leads to a very two-dimensional answer, follow up by asking

> Is he/she always like that? He/she sounds wonderful/terrible, but does he/she have any flaws/good traits?

Asking about how people see themselves can be tricky; don't be satisfied with "I don't know." Questions such as the following can be helpful:

> How do you think that others see you?
>
> Do you think that they think that they see you as basically the same over time, or as very changeable?

You will also want to get a sense of a person's capacity to mentalize by asking questions such as

> Tell me about a time when a person close to you disagreed with you. Why do you think he/she felt
> that way?

Learning about security

The following questions will help you to describe your patient's patterns of security in relationships:

> How do you feel when you're alone? Does it make you feel nervous or panicky?
>
> Are you still able to feel confident about your relationships when your loved ones aren't with you?
>
> Are you often worried that you will be left alone?
>
> Do you have close friends? How many, and for how long?
>
> Do you tend to stay in touch with old friends?
>
> Do you date (men, women, or both)? If so, how long do your relationships generally
> last?
>
> Do you tend to start relationships slowly or quickly?
>
> Do you tend to worry that the people you feel close to will leave you?
>
> Can other people soothe you when you are upset?

Learning about intimacy

About emotional intimacy:

> How do you think your friends/partners would describe the way you are with them?
>
> Would you describe yourself as relatively open emotionally?
>
> Are you comfortable telling your friends things about yourself that you're less than proud of?
>
> Is there someone whom you feel you can tell almost anything?
>
> Do you tend to push people away when you start to feel close?

About sexual intimacy:

> How many sexual partners do you have at any one time?
>
> Do you have sex as often as you'd like to? How often?
>
> Are you able/willing to initiate sex/to respond when your partner initiates it?

Are you generally more interested in sex early in a relationship? Later in a relationship?

How close do you feel to your partner during sex?

Does having sex with your partner make you feel closer or more distant from him/her?

Learning about mutuality in relationships

Since mutuality involves give and take, you can ask questions such as

Do you feel your partner/friend/parent gives you what you need?

Do you think your partner/friend/parent gets what he/she needs from you?

Describing relationships

Here's an example of how you might describe a person's relationship patterns:

*Although Mr M has **secure** relationships with each of his divorced parents and speaks to each of them every week, he has significant difficulty in his **relationships** with others. In particular, he has difficulty achieving **intimacy** in relationships, both with friends and romantic partners. After college, he became a loner and currently has only one close friend. He dated a few girls in high school and then had a long spell during which he had no relationships. His difficulties with intimacy are further illustrated by the fact that Mr M said that he was a virgin until several years ago when he had sex with a prostitute. He is frustrated by spending weekends alone and isolated in his apartment, playing his guitar and reading. His pattern of having intense crushes and then becoming quickly annoyed with his girlfriends' "neediness" suggests that he has a superficial **sense of self and other** and lacks **mutuality**. His early suspiciousness about the therapist's fees and policy of charging for missed sessions suggests that he might have difficulty with **trust**.*

Although Mr M has relatively secure relationships with his parents, he has trouble with both emotional and sexual intimacy with others. This has led to significant frustration and loneliness and has clearly impacted his function.

Variables for describing RELATIONSHIPS

Trust

Sense of self and other

Security

Intimacy

Mutuality

Suggested activity

What are the strengths and difficulties in these people's relationship patterns?

1. *Mr A is a 45-year-old divorced man who has joint custody of his two teenage daughters. "I'm happiest when they're with me," he explains, "I don't know what I'm going to do when they move out." He has had five or six relationships with women since separating from his wife 7 years ago and says that the women "start out nice but become needy in the end." He has a few male friends who live far away and with whom he rarely talks.*

Comment

Strengths: The fact that Mr A was able to marry and have children suggests a basic capacity to feel **secure** and to **trust** others. He continues to feel secure in his relationship with his teenagers.

Difficulties: Mr A's comment about his ex-wife points to trouble with his **sense of self and other**; he has to portray his wife as "all bad" while there must be some positive reason he chose to marry her and to have children with her. He speaks only of what he needs from his children, suggesting that he has difficulty with **mutuality**. His difficulty with **mutuality** is confirmed by what he says about girlfriends; he has trouble when they want more from him than he wants to give. He has some difficulty with **intimacy** since the relationships he has are relatively brief and his male friends live at a distance.

2. *Ms C is a 68-year-old woman whose husband of 40 years recently died. She describes him as "the love of my life" and says that they took care of each other in every way, adding, "It was almost like we were the same person." They had no children and few friends. She is very lonely now. She says she doesn't know how to make friends and sometimes sees no one for many days.*

Comment

Strengths: The length of Ms C's marriage and the closeness she felt to her husband of 40 years indicate her deep **trust** and **security** in that relationship. She also describes the relationship as quite **mutual**.

Difficulties: The intensity of Ms C's relationship with her husband, although positive, was also problematic for her. Her **sense of herself and other** was merged with her husband to the degree that she feels lost without him. Ms C's trouble making friends suggests that she has difficulty with **intimacy**.

6 Adapting

Key concepts

Every day, we have to adapt to internal and external stimulation
   Each person has his/her own

- thresholds for tolerating internal and external stimulation
- ways of adapting to internal and external stimulation

   We have many ways of adapting. They include

- defense mechanisms
- impulse control
- managing emotions
- sensory regulation

Life is not constant. Every day, we face different amounts of stimulation, both from outside and inside of us, that threaten our usual functioning. Some of this stimulation, such as the excitement of success, love, or joy, is welcome, while some, such as bad news, loss, or anxiety, is unwelcome. Overwhelming stimulation is sometimes called **stress** because it puts strain on the way we live our lives [36]. Thus, we all need ways to adapt to or manage both internal and external stimulation [37–41].

Defining the area: adapting

Adapting means adjusting. There are many types of internal and external stimulation that we need to adjust to on a daily basis:
   Internal stimulation includes

- thoughts and fantasies
- feelings and anxiety
- pain and other physical sensations

Psychodynamic Formulation, First Edition. Deborah L. Cabaniss, Sabrina Cherry, Carolyn J. Douglas, Ruth L. Graver, and Anna R. Schwartz.
© 2013 John Wiley & Sons, Ltd. Published 2013 by John Wiley & Sons, Ltd.

External stimulation includes

- relationships with others
- economic and work-related pressures
- trauma and other environmental events

Everyone has his/her own threshold for tolerating stimulation. Some people can tolerate high levels of affect, anxiety, and environmental stress, while others develop difficulties at much lower levels.

Variables for describing patterns of adapting

In the same way that all people have their own fingerprints, all people have their unique, characteristic ways of adapting to internal and external pressures [3, 18, 42–44]. We can describe these using the following four variables:

- defenses
- managing emotion
- impulse control
- stimulus regulation

Defenses

When we adapt to or manage stress, we keep the amount of excess stimulation at a level that allows us to continue functioning. We do this in many different ways, including blocking out feelings, filtering stimuli, forgetting things, or focusing our attention elsewhere. Sometimes we do these things purposefully and consciously, for example, when we say to ourselves, "I can't deal with this right now. I'm going to think about it later." Generally, however, we deal with stress without ever knowing that we are doing it. We call our unconscious ways of adapting to stress **defenses** [45–47]. Defenses function the way our sense of balance operates when we keep ourselves upright on the deck of a boat – automatically and continuously making tiny adjustments without our awareness. Just as our balance system automatically senses the tiny movements of the boat and deploys muscle movement to keep us upright, our mind senses tiny changes in our anxiety and emotional tone and deploys defenses to keep us functioning on an even keel.

As adults, we tend to use certain defenses on a regular basis. We can describe a person's characteristic defenses according to how

- adaptive
- flexible
- connected to thoughts and feelings

they are.

More and less adaptive defenses

Defenses can be classified in many ways. Since we are focusing on function, we have grouped them on a spectrum that relates to how well they help the person to adapt to stress while preserving function (see Table 6.1). **More adaptive defenses** preserve or enhance function; **less adaptive defenses** hinder function [48–50]. For example, if you're angry with your friend, **rationalizing** his/her behavior helps you to maintain the relationship, while **devaluing** him/her threatens it. Less adaptive defenses "work", that is, they decrease the awareness of a painful feeling, but at such a high cost that they impair function. Other examples of this are the use of **splitting** to handle strong opposing feelings at the cost of being able to have meaningful relationships, or **dissociating** to escape overwhelmingly bad feelings at the expense of being able to connect to reality [51].

Note that what is adaptive in one situation may not be in another. For example, if survival is at stake during wartime, it may be adaptive to use **denial** to stave off panic, but denial of a medical condition may preclude getting essential lifesaving care. Also, remember that people adapt to stress as well as they can in a given situation and that even less adaptive defenses developed because they were needed at some point in the person's life.

Let's think about whether Ms A's dominant defenses help or hinder her function:

> Ms A is a 45-year-old unemployed woman who comes for therapy because she is anxious, lonely, and isolated. She rapidly forms intense, close friendships, becomes disappointed when she perceives that friends are inattentive, and impulsively ends friendships. In the initial interview for therapy, she says to the therapist, "You understand me so well! Can we meet again tomorrow?"

Ms A tends to use **splitting**, as well as **idealization** and **devaluation**. Idealization allows Ms A to have relationships despite her anxiety, but sets up unrealistic expectations that destroy friendships before they can get off the ground. In addition, her tendency to split may make it difficult for her to keep jobs. Thus, her defensive strategy is not particularly adaptive.

Flexibility

No matter how good a strategy is for adapting to stress, it can't work in every situation. Consequently, people need to be **flexible** enough to use a range of adaptive strategies. People without defensive flexibility often seem controlling, difficult, or brittle. Think of the person who always has to win an argument, or who always manages stress by making jokes – even when they're not appropriate. In addition, while a certain defense may work well at a particular time of life, the same strategy may become a hindrance at a later point.

Example

> Ms B is a 40-year-old woman with tremendous anxiety, which she handles by being extremely organized and limiting the amount of novelty in her life. While this strategy worked for her when she was a single woman, it is now impeding her children's social schedules, her family's vacation options, and her husband's leisure activities. Although her friends tell her to "just ease up," she is unable to change her patterns.

Ms B's defensive strategy, while helpful for keeping her anxiety within tolerable bounds, is overly rigid and is having a negative impact on her relationships.

Table 6.1 Defense mechanisms

Defense	Definition
Less adaptive	
Splitting	Keeping good and bad feelings separate in order to protect the good (*Ms A experienced her abusive mother as all good and her sister as all bad.*)
Projection	Perceiving unacceptable qualities or feelings as originating outside of the self (*Mr B worried that his friend did not like him when actually he did not like his friend.*)
Projective identification	Projecting a thought or feeling into another person, then interacting with that person to make him/her experience the projected feeling (*Ms C is unaware of her anger at her boyfriend; she is then one hour late to their date, making him angry with her.*)
Pathological idealization and devaluation	Attributing overly positive or negative feelings to others (*At his first therapy session, Mr D tells his therapist, "You are clearly the best therapist in the city. Much better than my last therapist, who was an idiot."*)
Denial	Disavowing unacceptable feelings and thoughts (*Ms E, who has frequent seizures from alcohol withdrawal, says that she does not have a drinking problem.*)
Dissociation	Disconnecting unacceptable thoughts and feelings from current reality (*Mr F had no memory of being yelled at by his boss.*)
Acting out	Expressing unacceptable thoughts or feelings in actions (*After a difficult therapy session, Ms G ate a gallon of ice cream.*)
Regression	Using coping strategies from earlier periods of development to deal with stressful events or feelings (*During exam week, Mr H stopped showering and cleaning his room.*)
More adaptive	
Isolation of affect	Forgetting a feeling while remaining conscious of the associated thought (*Ms I said that she had no feelings about having been left by her husband.*)
Intellectualization	Replacing painful or uncomfortable feelings with excessive thinking (*Mr J dealt with his cancer diagnosis by focusing on extensive research data about the disease.*)
Rationalization	Explaining unacceptable behavior or feelings in a logical manner (*Ms K said that she was glad that she was fired because she never liked her job.*)
Displacement	Redirecting feelings or impulses to other people or activities (*Unaware of his anger at his wife, Mr L explodes at his son.*)
Somatization	Experiencing uncomfortable feelings or thoughts as physical symptoms (*After her bad review, Ms M develops a headache and takes a sick day.*)

Table 6.1 *(continued)*

Defense	Definition
Undoing	"Fixing" unacceptable thoughts or feelings or behavior by opposing behaviors (*Ms N treats her best friend badly and then buys her an especially nice birthday present.*)
Reaction formation	Reversing an unacceptable feeling by experiencing it as its opposite (*Irritated by his toddler, Mr O becomes overprotective.*)
Excessive emotionality	Forgetting a thought while remaining aware of the associated feeling (*Unable to acknowledge his ambivalence about getting married, Mr P was anxious and irritable during the entire wedding planning process.*)
Identification	Striving to be like another person to deal with jealous or competitive feelings (*Ms Q gradually began to dress exactly like her more popular roommate.*)
Externalization	Perceiving internal conflicts or experiences as arising from external circumstances (*Mr R blames his tenuous position at work for making him feel unsure of himself.*)
Sexualization	Expressing uncomfortable thoughts or feelings as flirtatiousness or overly sexual behaviors (*Anxious about a job interview, Ms S dresses inappropriately in overly revealing clothing.*)
Repression	Keeping uncomfortable thoughts, feelings, and fantasies from conscious awareness (*After an unpleasant therapy session, Ms T forgets to come to her next appointment.*)
Turning against the self	Blaming oneself rather than experiencing unacceptable feelings toward another person (*Mr U blamed himself when his irritable mother stopped talking to him.*)
Most adaptive	
Humor	Expressing uncomfortable thoughts or feelings as jokes (*After she was left by her fiancé at the altar, Ms V said, "I knew we should have chosen another caterer."*)
Altruism	Turning painful feelings into doing for others (*After his father died of cancer, Mr W finds comfort in starting a foundation to provide support for patients with cancer and their families.*)
Sublimation	Converting unacceptable impulses into more useful forms (*When sad, Ms X makes startlingly beautiful, mournful paintings.*)
Suppression	Consciously deciding not to focus on difficult thoughts or feelings (*Faced with a deadline at work, Mr Y decides not to focus on an ongoing conflict he is having with his family.*)

Adapted from Gabbard [47]

How defenses deal with thoughts and feelings

Some defenses work by keeping stressful **feelings** out of awareness, while others work by keeping stressful **thoughts** out of awareness. Consider the way two men deal with the stress of their recent divorces:

> *Mr C says that it is a good time to divorce because property values are high and it will be easy to sell the house.*

> *Three weeks after his divorce, Mr D became extremely anxious about a mole on his leg and began racing around to dermatologists for different opinions.*

Mr C uses **rationalization**, which allows him to keep his feelings out of awareness while remaining aware of his thoughts. Mr D uses **somatization**, which keeps his anxious feelings conscious but his thoughts about the divorce out of awareness. People who tend to use defenses that keep *feelings* out of awareness are sometimes said to have an **obsessive** defensive style, while people who tend to use defenses that keep *thoughts* out of awareness are sometimes said to have a **hysterical** defensive style [52].

Managing emotions

The excitement of taking your first steps, the pride of graduating from college, the joy of watching your child being born – without these feelings, life would be colorless. It's also important to be able to experience more difficult feelings, such as sadness, loss, and disappointment. They help us to understand ourselves and others – without them we would have trouble learning from experience, feeling empathy, and having relationships. Feelings also motivate us and give us "zest" for life. Some people are more able to experience, tolerate, and express a wide range of feelings than others, as in these examples:

> Mr E   *I just love being with my grandchildren. They're so full of life! Just watching them go back and forth on the swing takes my breath away. I can't wait to see them again!*

> Mr F   *We spent the day with the grandchildren. We had lunch. My daughter has her hands full. Guess we'll see them again in a few weeks.*

Two grandfathers, two different experiences. Mr E is full of feeling – you can almost hear the excitement in his voice. Mr F sounds flatter, less feeling-filled. Noting whether the person has a range of feelings is also important – it can't be all good or all bad.

While it's important to be able to experience feelings, it's also important to be able to manage them. Out-of-control feelings – whether they're positive or negative – can be overwhelming and stressful. Every individual has a different capacity to tolerate feelings, including anxiety. For example, consider Ms G and Ms H:

As she listened to her boyfriend breaking up with her, Ms G began to feel out of control. She started to scream uncontrollably, then went to the cabinet and began breaking plates.

As she listened to her boyfriend breaking up with her, Ms H felt many feelings. She sat quietly and waited for him to finish. She knew that she could not respond right away without getting very upset. She told him that she needed to leave, drove home, and took a hot bath. Later that evening, she cried as she told the story to her roommate. They made dinner together and watched a movie.

While they were both upset, Ms H could manage her feelings and keep herself reasonably calm, while Ms G could not.

Note that people may have difficulty managing emotions either because they have trouble handling even small amounts of anxiety or emotions or because they are overwhelmed by chronic anxiety and mood symptoms.

Impulse control

Impulses come in many forms. People with difficulty controlling impulses can have trouble with

- managing appetites (substances, food, sex)
- gambling
- controlling aggression/violence
- stealing

Consider these two impulsive people:

Mr I loves to eat. He is quite obese and his cholesterol is too high. He wakes up every day saying, "I'm going on a diet today," but by 7 pm he's tearing through his cabinets and freezer, looking for cookies and ice cream. He often eats in secret so that his family is not aware of how much he is eating. He goes to sleep feeling defeated every night.

Ms J has a hard time not speaking in class. She always feels that she has something really interesting to say, and she always has her hand in the air. In her last class evaluation, her professor suggested that she might want to "give some of her classmates some air time," but even when she tries to stay quiet the words just seem to "pop out."

Being impulsive isn't necessarily always bad. Sometimes, being overly controlled can be problematic. The person who is unable to do anything spontaneous – from buying a new pair of shoes to agreeing to an impromptu gathering after work – often has difficulties in relationships with others. Similarly, risk-taking, which is inversely related to impulse control, can lead to self-destructive behavior but can also be essential for large-scale business moves. For some, risk-taking activities, like bungee jumping and scuba diving in caves, is pleasurable, while for others it is terrifying.

People control their impulses in many ways. They learn to slow down, delay gratification, and count to 10. Some can do it on their own, but others need the support of 12-step programs or religious beliefs. Understanding and describing a person's successful strategies for controlling himself/herself is as important as documenting his/her struggles with impulse control – again, remember your patients' strengths as well as their difficulties.

Sensory regulation

Noise, smells, textures – these stimuli are everywhere and we need to be able to adjust to them. As with the other types of stimuli we have discussed, people vary widely in their ability to tolerate and adapt to these sensations. Some people startle easily when they hear a telephone ring, or become nauseated if they sense a whiff of a bad odor; others are oblivious. Some people enjoy very stimulating environments, like rock concerts or Times Square on New Year's Eve; others are bothered when the sounds of children playing disturb them during walks in the park. Difficulty adjusting to sensory stimuli can be a major impediment to functioning. Consider Ms K:

> Ms K is unable to use public transportation of any type, including air travel, because of her intolerance of the way other people smell. While this is a particular problem on subways and buses, she cannot tolerate the faintest whiff of another person's smell, including perfume. This has caused her difficulties at work and play since she has not been able to attend important out-of-town conferences or travel to family gatherings.

Ms K's inability to adapt to sensory stimulation is disrupting her function and is thus an important aspect of her capacity to adapt.

Learning about how someone adapts

Learning about defenses

Here are some questions that can help you learn about your patients' defensive style:

> What's your sense of how you react to anxiety and strong feelings? Would others agree?
>
> Do you feel you always react in the same way, or do you feel you have different strategies depending on the circumstances?

Here are some questions you can ask yourself that can help you answer these questions:

> Does this person tend to use splitting as a dominant defense?

Does this person's defensive style seem to get in the way of his/her interpersonal relationships?

If you offer alternative ways of looking at things, is the person flexible or unable to shift perspective?

In talking to you, does the person use many feeling-filled words?

Does what the person say seem dry or devoid of feelings, even when he/she is talking about something painful or exciting?

When talking about something painful, does the person show his/her feelings? Does he/she offer an explanation/excuse for the feelings?

Do you feel caught up in the patient's dramatic storytelling? Or do you feel bored and detached from what the person is saying?

Learning about impulse control

Many clinicians ask about substance use and eating disorders, but learning about impulse control and judgment involves much more than that. We want to be able to describe the kinds of problems that people have with impulses, but we also want to describe the individual ways they try to curb impulses. Questions like the following can be helpful:

Do you think that people would describe you as a risk-taker?

Do you ever feel that you're too impulsive?

Would someone describe you as having a quick temper?

Do you tend to hang back or just jump into things?

Do you find it hard to keep from doing things you think you probably shouldn't do?

Do you ever drink/eat to excess? If so, how much?

What types of things do you do to keep yourself from being impulsive?

Learning about managing emotions

What happens when you get angry or anxious? Can you "sit" with the feeling or do you feel driven to do something? If so, what?

Would people describe you as calm and even-tempered? As volatile?

Do you ever become physically violent with others? What happens?

Learning about sensory regulation

Do you think that you're particularly sensitive to things like loud noises or smells?

Do you ever experience the environment in ways that you think that others don't?

Describing adapting

Here is how we might describe someone's capacity to adapt using the variables we have outlined:

> Ms L's ability to **adapt** is a major strength. Chronically ill with rheumatoid arthritis since childhood, she uses highly adaptive **defenses** to deal with stress. For example, she runs a foundation for children with rheumatoid arthritis that raises millions of dollars a year and gives her significant satisfaction (sublimation), and when people stop her on the street and comment on her use of a cane at such a young age, she often uses humor to deflect the confrontation. In highly stressful situations, she can cry and become dramatic, using defenses that tend to **emphasize emotions**. Her range of defenses is fairly **flexible**. If anything, her **impulse control** is too good – she loathes taking chances and this has sometimes led her to miss opportunities.

This description takes into consideration both types of defenses that Ms L uses, as well as their flexibility and the way they handle thoughts and feelings. It also considers her impulse control.

From here, we'll move on to consider cognition, our fourth area of functioning.

Variables for describing ADAPTING

Defense mechanisms

    more adaptive/less adaptive

    flexibility

    connection to thoughts and feelings

Impulse control

Managing emotions

Sensory regulation

Suggested activity

How would you describe Mr A's patterns of adapting?

> Mr A, a 65-year-old man, has just been told that he has prostate cancer. He begins complaining of headaches and toothaches and constantly shuttles back and forth to doctors and dentists. He is irritable and tells everyone he knows how frightened he is. His incessant phone calls lead his friends to begin to avoid him. In order to try to take his mind off his impending treatment, his wife tries to engage him in refinishing their dining room table, which he has wanted to do for many years, but he is unable to refocus. She is becoming increasingly exasperated with him and says that this is exactly how he behaved when their son had trouble with drugs many years before.

Comment

Mr A's primary defense is **somatization**. This defensive strategy, which leads him to overuse medical and dental care and threatens his relationships, is not particularly adaptive. His inability to shift coping strategies during the current crisis, as well as the similarity between his current mechanisms and those he employed many years ago, suggest that his patterns for dealing with stress are quite **inflexible**. He also has difficulty **managing his emotions**, and has **poor impulse control**, as evidenced by his inability to restrain himself from calling friends repeatedly. Finally, his preoccupation with minor physical pain may reflect impaired **stimulus regulation**.

7 Cognition

Key concepts

The way people think is central to the way they function.
  We can describe cognitive function using the following variables:

- general cognitive abilities
- decision making and problem solving
- self-reflection and reality testing
- mentalization
- judgment

Defining the area: cognition

Cogito ergo sum – Descartes famously asserted that the fact that we think is evidence of our existence [53]. The way we think is reflected in almost everything that we do, including problem solving, organizing our thoughts, remembering things, and focusing our attention. Some people have strengths in one area of cognitive function but difficulties in another – consider the absent-minded professor who, while being a brilliant lecturer, is disorganized and always late to appointments. Rather than placing a value on one type of thinking over another, we want to describe all of the ways in which people think and to determine how adaptive they are.

Being able to describe someone's cognitive function is essential to the process of constructing a psychodynamic formulation for several reasons. First, the way we think is key to our function, and thus, we want to be able to hypothesize about its development. Second, the way we think can affect other aspects of our development. For example, when children have problems with attention or organization, it may affect the way they perceive themselves (self-esteem) and how they are viewed and treated by teachers and peers at school (relationships with others). Finally, since cognitive functions develop and change over the course of a person's lifetime (see Part Three), carefully observing and describing problems in this area can give us clues as to when problems may have occurred for an individual during development.

Psychodynamic Formulation, First Edition. Deborah L. Cabaniss, Sabrina Cherry, Carolyn J. Douglas, Ruth L. Graver, and Anna R. Schwartz.

Variables for describing cognition

Reviewing the wide range of cognitive functions is beyond the scope of this book. However, we can think of some general clusters of cognitive functions that are essential to describe. They are

- general cognitive abilities
- decision making and problem solving
- capacity for self-reflection and reality testing
- mentalization
- judgment

General cognitive ability

How smart is he? Why does she keep forgetting things? Why can't he keep track of his homework? As therapists, these are questions we ask ourselves about our patients every day, and they relate to our patients' general cognitive abilities (see Table 7.1). While assessing these areas of function sometimes requires formal testing (e.g., intelligence, memory, attention) [54], we can and should make comments about general function in these areas, particularly when they represent clear strengths or difficulties:

Examples

Ms A started winning science contests in the third grade. She had her first patent in college and was awarded tenure at MIT at age 28.

Mr B presents with difficulty staying focused on tasks at work. He says that he could never focus on homework and had to repeat 2nd grade twice.

Ms C, who is CEO of her own company, comes to every session having forgotten something – her keys, your check, her umbrella. "It drives my husband crazy," she says, "I remember everything at work, but in my personal life – forget it!"

Mr D, who was a professor in his home country, immigrated to the United States at age 60 and has never felt fully comfortable communicating in English.

The cognitive function of these individuals will affect their functioning in every other area – the way they think about themselves, their relationships with others, how they adapt to stress, and their work and play. This is true for all of us, but is particularly significant when cognitive function represents a major strength or difficulty.

Table 7.1 General cognitive abilities

intelligence
memory
attention
speech and language

Decision making and problem solving

People make decisions and solve problems in very different ways. Think about the variety of methods that people use when choosing a new car:

> *Mr E buys a Buick because that's the car his father always drove.*
>
> *Mr F goes into the first dealership he sees and buys a car off the lot.*
>
> *Mr G chooses his car because of the color.*
>
> *Mr H reads 3 years' worth of Consumer Reports articles about cars, test drives five models, creates a rating system, and ultimately buys the car that gets the most points according to his scale.*

All of these people have the capacity to make decisions, but their decision making processes are vastly different. People vary widely in the way they make decisions. Some people are very detail oriented, while others are more impressionistic; some people make decisions based on research, while others are guided by "hunches." Some people are planners, and some "take things as they come." Still others have considerable creative talents that help them not only with solving problems but also with everything from inventing new recipes to making scientific discoveries. Consider the way Ms I and Ms J plan their parties:

> *Ms I is having a party. She creates a list of things that she needs to do and checks them off as she goes. A week before the party, the caterer calls and tells her that she has broken her leg and will not be able to do the job. Ms I pulls out the list of caterers that she originally considered and begins calling them until she finds one who is available.*
>
> *Ms J is having a party. She changes her mind five times about the theme and the type of food to serve. She doodles "things to do" on the backs of napkins and then never refers to them. When she goes to the bakery the night before and finds out that they are sold out of the desserts she wanted, she turns on her favorite music and bakes all night.*

Ms I is organized, attends to details, thinks ahead, and is able to problem solve in a calm manner. On the contrary, Ms J is more spontaneous, frequently changes her mind, and solves problems in an emotional way. Ultimately, both parties could be great successes, but the thought process that went into planning them would have been quite different. Our job is not to judge which is better, but to describe our patients' problem solving styles and to think about how they positively or negatively impact function.

Problem solving requires the ability to organize thinking, plan ahead, and think creatively (see Table 7.2). As with general cognitive abilities, these capacities can have a major impact on the development of other functions as well.

Example

> *Ms K, an 18-year-old college sophomore, comes to her session saying that all of her friends "hate" her. "They put me in charge of signing up for the housing lottery and I screwed the whole thing up. It's so confusing! I knew that it was coming up but couldn't get it together to get all the papers in, see the rooms – I just couldn't cope. What am I going to do?"*

Ms K's inability to organize this project and to problem solve creatively has clearly gotten in the way of her relationships, and this is probably not the first time that something like this has happened to her.

Table 7.2 Problem solving abilities

decision making
problem solving
organizing thoughts
planning
creative thinking

Self-reflection

Another important aspect of thinking is the capacity to examine one's own thoughts and behaviors. This is called **self-reflection** [55]. Some people do this naturally, asking themselves questions like, "I wonder why I said/did that?" while others are more likely to say, "It is what it is," and go no further. Self-reflection is the ability to step back, sometimes just a little bit, from one's experience in order to try to understand it. **Psychological mindedness** [55], which is related to self-reflection, is the ability to think about possible unconscious motivations for one's thoughts, feelings, and behavior. Being able to self-reflect helps people to learn about and improve their feelings about themselves and their relationships with others. For example, consider Mr L:

> The week before Valentine's Day, Mr L and M, his girlfriend of 1 year, walk past a flower shop. As they pass, his girlfriend says, "Yellow roses are my favorite." On Valentine's Day, Mr L gets M a card. Later that night, M starts to cry and says, "I thought that you were going to buy me roses!" Mr L is mystified and says, "Why would you think that?" When he buys M a card for her birthday 2 months later, she breaks up with him. Mr L feels blindsided, telling his therapist, "You can't get it right with women."

Unable to be self-reflective, Mr L does not ask himself how he might have contributed to the situation.

The capacity for reflection is also related to **reality testing** [55]. Reality testing is the ability to differentiate reality from fantasy. Needless to say, it is essential for every aspect of function, from relationships to work. Some people intermittently lose the capacity to test reality during periods of stress. Still others can test reality but sometimes doubt their conclusions.

Examples

> Ms N is sure that her boss is out to fire her because, "He found out that I have special powers and feels threatened."

> Ms O says, "I know that my husband is faithful, but when I get mad I always start thinking that he's having an affair. At those moments, I have difficulty getting perspective on that."

While Ms N is frankly unable to test reality, Ms O has intermittent difficulty with this. Both issues are important to note and to describe.

Mentalization

Mentalization (see Chapters 5 and 10) is the capacity to understand that other people have thoughts and feelings that are different from one's own [56]. The ability to mentalize is central to the ability to empathize with others. Consider the difference between Ms P and Ms Q:

> When her therapist is uncharacteristically 10 minutes late to a session, Ms P says, "How could you do this to me! You know my LSAT's are tomorrow and I'm crazy with anxiety! What were you thinking?"

> When her therapist is uncharacteristically 10 minutes late to a session, Ms Q says, "Hi – that's so weird that you're late – you never are. I hope that everything is OK. I wonder if you had an emergency. It can't be easy to be a therapist."

Ms P can't imagine that things could be going on in the mind and life of her therapist that don't relate to her, while Ms Q can. Being able to describe this ability is important for understanding cognitive function.

Judgment

The capacity to consider the consequences of behavior, often called **judgment** [55], is another cognitive function. Judgment involves not only being aware of the appropriateness and likely consequences of an intended behavior but also behaving in a way that reflects this awareness. In psychodynamic terms, the capacity to know right from wrong is part of **superego function** [55]. As with many of the other cognitive functions outlined, judgment is not an "on or off" function, but rather can wax and wane in different circumstances.

Examples

Mr R is usually a very responsible father, but when he is drunk he often forgets to pick his children up from school.

Ms S knows that she should use a condom when having sex with a new partner, but says that she sometimes "gets caught up in the moment."

These people "know" the right thing to do and even have a sense of the consequences of their behavior, but sometimes do not act on them. People's judgment can have an enormous impact on every aspect of their functioning and is thus important to describe.

Learning about cognition

Learning about general cognitive function

Information about general cognitive function will come from your direct experience with people. You can notice things like

When they tell their story, is it organized in a coherent way?

Are they able to remember appointments and plan for new ones?

Do they come to appointments and pay bills on time?

Do they have a reasonable fund of knowledge?

You can also ask direct questions, such as

Are you someone who is usually on time or are you often late?

At your job/school are you generally able to concentrate and get your work done?

Are you generally well organized? Disorganized?

If your evaluation suggests significant problems in general cognitive function, you may want to consider administering a brief cognitive screening test, such as the Mini-Mental Status Examination (MMSE) [54], or referring the patient for neuropsychological testing. The presence of cognitive problems in association with other psychiatric disorders such as depression or anxiety should lead you to consider the potential impact of these disorders on cognition.

Learning about decision making and problem solving

You will often learn about this from the chief complaint or from the way a person finds time to meet or decides about starting treatment. You can also ask direct questions about this, such as

Do you find it easy/hard to make decisions?

Tell me about a recent decision that you made. How did you reach it?

Do you typically research options or do you tend to "trust your gut?"

When you have many things to do, do you make a list?

Learning about self-reflection

A good way to assess self-reflection is by trial interpretation. Consider the following exchange between Ms T and her therapist:

Ms T   *I can't believe I slept through my sister's baby shower! I was so tired. I think my alarm clock must have malfunctioned.*

Therapist   *Well, last time you were talking about how hard it is for you that your sister is having a baby when your relationship with your boyfriend has just ended. Do you think maybe you didn't want to go to the shower?*

Ms T   *Wow, are you saying I overslept on purpose? That does kind of sound like me. I really didn't want to go. She doesn't even ask me how I'm doing.*

Psychological mindedness does not mean understanding everything right away. While Ms T does not immediately consider that she might be ambivalent about her sister, she is receptive and thoughtful when the therapist asks her to consider possible unconscious motivations. Ms T is reasonably psychologically minded and self-reflective. A less psychologically minded person might have replied to the therapist's comments by saying, *"No way! Of course I'm happy for her. Therapists always think there's double meaning in everything."*

Learning about mentalization

A good way to assess mentalization is to ask the patient to think about how another person thinks or feels, as in this example:

Ms U	*I'm so mad at my friend Jane – she hasn't responded to my last phone call and I'm sure it's because she's angry at me.*
Therapist	*When did you call her?*
Ms U	*About 20 minutes ago.*
Therapist	*Do you think that there could be another reason why she hasn't called back yet?*
Ms U	*No – if people like you, they get back to you right away.*

Ms U's inability to think of another reason for her friend's behavior suggests that she has problems with mentalizing. Asking people questions like

> *Do you think that he/she could be looking at things differently?*
> *How do you imagine that I might be feeling?*

can help you to gauge their ability to mentalize.

Learning about judgment

To assess judgment, consider asking questions like the following:

> *Are you a person who tends to follow rules?*
> *Have there been times when you broke rules? How did you decide to do that?*
> *Would people who know you describe you as someone with good judgment?*

As always, listening to stories can help here. Stories about poor investments, rule bending, failure to use condoms and other methods of birth control, and driving while intoxicated can tell you a great deal about a person's judgment. If you think that a story clearly illustrates impaired judgment, find out whether the person thinks that he/she acted wisely. This can help you to differentiate judgment from impulse control. For example, consider this exchange:

Patient #1 *So I met this guy at a bar and we went back to his place and had sex.*

Therapist *Did you use a condom?*

Patient #1 *No.*

Therapist *Was that what you meant to do?*

Patient #1 *Yeah, it's fine. Plus, guys hate condoms.*

This patient clearly used bad judgment. On the other hand, consider another patient's response to the same question

Patient #2 *No, are you kidding? It's so dangerous – but in the moment I just can't stop to make sure that I'm safe – I just act.*

This patient knows the right thing to do but shows poor impulse control. Judgment is still impaired, but the difference is important for the treatment.

Describing patterns related to cognition

Here is an example of how you might describe patterns of cognition in a psychodynamic formulation:

*Ms V seems to have good **general cognitive function**. She arrived on time for her evaluation sessions and immediately began to tell her life story in a fluid, coherent way. She is capable of **making decisions, problem solving**, and exercising good **judgment**, as evidenced by her recent ability to choose and buy her own apartment, despite last-minute difficulties with the closing. Her capacity for **self-reflection** seems to be a strength. When the therapist pointed out to her that her description of her childhood as "happy" did not entirely fit with what she said about her mother's alcoholism and angry outbursts, she said, "That's an interesting comment. I never thought about that." Despite these strengths, she seems to have difficulty with **mentalization** since she could not imagine that her recent affair might have contributed to her husband's decision to leave her.*

Finally, we'll address our last area of functioning – work and play – in Chapter 8.

Variables for describing COGNITION

General cognitive abilities

Problem solving abilities

Capacity for self-reflection

Mentalization

Judgment

Suggested activity

How would you describe the cognitive function of these patients?

Mr A, a talented 35-year-old interior designer, was doing very well at work until he was promoted to manage others. He is now alternately angry and anxious and is unable to keep track of what the members of his team are doing. He has difficulty delegating work and ends up redoing much of what they do. He dreads the weekly meeting when he has to report to his boss – the first time he walked in with 10 lists that ended up scattered all over the floor.

Ms B says that she is "fed up" with her husband because he spends too much time at work. He has a high-profile job at a bank that pays for their lavish lifestyle, which Ms B enjoys. "Our marital problems are all due to the fact that he's a workaholic," she says, "The only way for things to get better is for him to just say NO the next time his boss tells him to stay late!"

Comment

Mr A seems to have **creative talent**; however, he lacks **organizational abilities**. He also has difficulty **making decisions**, particularly relating to managing his team. Ms B is unable to **mentalize** and lacks capacity for **self-reflection**.

8 Work and Play

Key concepts

People spend most of their lives engaged in some type of work or play.
   Describing whether people's work and play are

- well matched to their developmental level/talents/limitations
- comfortable/satisfying for them
- adequate for care of self and dependents
- culturally sanctioned

helps us to understand their function in this area.

People spend their time doing myriad things. They work and study; they relax and socialize. As mental health professionals, we don't have preconceived notions about what people *should* do in life, but we are interested in assessing whether what they *choose* to do is well suited for their lives as individuals and as members of society. In order to do this, we have to be able to describe what people spend their time doing. Freud is reputed to have said that people need to be able to "love and work" [57], and to this many have added "play" [58, 59]. Having discussed "love" (relationships) in Chapter 5, let's now think about work and play.

Defining the area: work and play

Work

Webster's dictionary defines **work** as "physical or mental effort exerted to do or make something; purposeful activity" [60]. Unless they are completely mentally and physically incapacitated, most people in the world are engaged in some type of work. Although we generally think about work as something that someone does to earn money, there are all kinds of work. Work can be the following:

- **For money or not for money** – A 2nd grader's work is going to school, and a stay-at-home parent's work is taking care of children. People who volunteer their services are still doing work.

Psychodynamic Formulation, First Edition. Deborah L. Cabaniss, Sabrina Cherry, Carolyn J. Douglas, Ruth L. Graver, and Anna R. Schwartz.
© 2013 John Wiley & Sons, Ltd. Published 2013 by John Wiley & Sons, Ltd.

- **Consistent or sporadic** – Two girls might both work as babysitters, but if one works every weekend and the other one only works now and then, their work patterns are very different.

- **In the home or out of the home** – Again, it's important to remember that a great deal of work happens within the home, including cleaning, cooking, child-rearing, and taking care of elders.

- **Skilled or unskilled** – Some work can be done with very little instruction, while other work requires extensive training. Note that training can take many forms, including technical schools, graduate schools, and apprenticeships.

Play

Relaxing on a beach, watching TV, reading fiction, socializing, throwing a football, traveling, cooking – everyone has a different way of playing. People who know how to play may have healthier emotional lives and may age more successfully [61, 62]. As mental health professionals, we often forget to ask about what people do to relax, but patterns of play are central to a person's function. When thinking about play, consider the following:

- **How much time it occupies in the person's life** – Two people might say that they enjoy reading, but if one reads a few magazines a month and the other goes to two book clubs per week, they have different patterns of play.

- **Whether they play alone or with others** – Some people enjoy solitary forms of relaxation, such as building models in the basement, while others enjoy going to huge rock concerts or throwing weekly dinner parties.

- **Depth and breadth of their involvement** – Some people are very involved in only one form of play, while others try many. For example, one person might cite sailing as her only leisure activity, but does it intensely; in contrast, another person might cite numerous pastimes but engages in them superficially.

- **Sex as play** – Sex can be an important aspect of the way people relax and enjoy themselves. Sexual activity has also been shown to be important to an adult's mental and emotional health [63]. It is important to ask about this part of our patients' lives, including whether they regularly engage in sexual activity, whether it is satisfying, with whom they are sexually active, and whether it is in the context of a loving relationship.

- **Absence of play** – If people do not mention any leisure activity, be sure to ask. It's crucial to find out whether there's something that the person enjoys doing – even if it's watching TV or reading the newspaper. Some people, however, have no leisure activities, indicating that they have tremendous difficulty relaxing and enjoying themselves.

Variables for describing work and play

Along with describing *what* a person does for work and play, we also want to think about *how well suited* these patterns are for the person's life as an individual and as a member of society. To do this, we can consider whether the person's work and play patterns are

- well matched to developmental level/talents/limitations
- comfortable/satisfying/pleasurable
- adequate for care of self and dependents
- culturally sanctioned

Are work and play well matched to developmental level, training, talents, and limitations?

A 16-year-old who works in a fast-food restaurant to make extra money during high school may be highly motivated, but a 45-year-old chemist with a PhD in the same job is underemployed. A 12-year-old boy who plays video games on the weekends with his friends is having developmentally appropriate fun, but a 55-year-old man who plays video games all day at work may jeopardize his job. When thinking about work and play, we not only have to think about what the person is doing, but whether it matches the person's developmental phase, training, talents, and limitations.

Example

Ms A, a 35-year-old woman, spent 7 years getting her PhD in English. She won a prize for her thesis and was offered a tenure-track position at a nearby college. She began that position, but left after 6 months, saying that she did not like the pressure of academia. For the past 5 years, she has worked as a fact checker at a small magazine.

Given her training, we would describe Ms A's work as poorly matched to her level of training.

Are work and play comfortable and pleasurable?

Fun is not just for kids – everyone needs to do things that they enjoy. Some people love their work, while for others it is simply something that they have to do to put food on the table. Work can also be satisfying but not necessarily enjoyable. Interestingly, some people do not find their leisure activities pleasurable – consider the person who hates camping but is constantly dragged into the woods by his/her partner, or a son who hates golf but feels compelled to play with his father every weekend.

Example

Mr B is a 40-year-old man who runs 20 miles a day. This has caused him myriad injuries and he becomes nauseated each day before he begins his run. Mr B was a track and field star in college, and he feels compelled to continue this regimen to fend off aging.

Although Mr B may once have enjoyed this level of exercise, it has become compulsive and has ceased to give him pleasure.

Are work and play adequate for care of self and dependents?

People may love their work, but it may not pay the bills. Consider the writer who is enjoying creating his novel but can't pay for health insurance. For some people, making a lot of money is not a high priority, but they still have to have enough money to pay for basic expenses of living, including food, shelter, and health care, for themselves and their dependents. Sometimes, a person is supported by a spouse or other family members. In this situation, it's important to assess whether this is a mutually agreed upon situation and if it is satisfactory to the individual. Here are two different examples of this situation:

Mr C never liked his job, while his wife is very gratified by her career. When they had children, they decided that Mr C would stay home, while his wife would continue to work outside the home to support the family financially.

In this situation, Mr C's individual work does not allow him to care for himself, but he is in a mutually agreed upon financial situation in which his wife supports the family.

Ms D, a 35-year-old graduate student, receives monthly checks from her father to cover her rent. This has strained their relationship and makes her feel like "a kid."

In this situation, Ms D's inability to support herself is leading to problems in her experience of herself and her relationship with others.

Play is also important with regard to self-care, since regular physical exercise is essential for physical and mental health [64]. If a person is unable to exercise, for example because she has to work three jobs in order to feed her family, then her pattern of play is inadequate to care for herself.

Are work and play culturally sanctioned?

In order to fully understand a person's work and play patterns, it's important to know whether they fit into the world in which the person lives. For example, if people make their living through illegal activities, or if their leisure involves harming others or using illicit substances, then it's hard to say that their work and play patterns are well suited to life in their environment.

Example

Ms E, a 29-year-old woman who works as a teacher, says that every night after work she goes home and drinks close to a bottle of wine. She says that it's the only way she can relax after a hard day at work.

Although Ms E is happy with this leisure activity, it is problematic because it involves abuse of a substance.

Aside from work and leisure activities that involve substance abuse and frankly illegal activities, thinking about whether work and play patterns are culturally sanctioned can be tricky, particularly in cross-cultural situations. Consider the following examples:

Mr F immigrated to the United States from a country in which it is typical for men to work extremely long hours, precluding their ability to attend their children's athletic events. When Mr F fails to come to any of his son's basketball games for 2 years, the coach calls to ask whether there is a problem at home.

In this case, Mr F's work schedule might be typical for one environment, but is seemingly problematic for another.

Ms G tells her therapist that she and her husband spend every weekend with her parents. When the therapist wonders if this makes Ms G feel dependent, Ms G explains that this is what all of her friends from "the old neighborhood" do.

Again, understanding Ms G's pattern of leisure requires sensitivity to her cultural background.

Learning about work and play

Learning about whether work and play are well matched to developmental level, talents, and limitations

For people who are working:

How long have you been doing the work you do?

Did this work require training? If so what kind?

If the person is trained to do one thing and is doing another, why is that?

For students:

How did you choose what and where you are studying?

Does this course of study seem like a good intellectual fit?

Are you working toward something, such as a career?

For play:

When did you begin this leisure activity?

Do you play with people your age?

How much time does it take up in your life?

How does it fit in with other things that you do in your life?

Learning about whether work and play are comfortable and pleasurable

How do you like your work? Is it hard to go to work in the morning?

Do you find your work satisfying? Are there things about it that you find more or less enjoyable than others?

Are there things that you look forward to doing?

Do you have fun? If so, doing what?

Learning about whether work and play are adequate for care of self and dependents

Are you able to make ends meet? For yourself? For your family?

Are you satisfied with the way in which you support yourself financially?

Do you receive financial help from someone else (including the government)? How do you feel about this? Are you in debt?

Are you able to get regular physical exercise? If not, why?

Learning about whether work and play patterns are culturally sanctioned

Have you ever been in trouble with the law? For what type of activity?

Do your leisure activities ever involve illicit substances?

Are you ever concerned that something that you're doing might not be legal?

Describing work and play patterns

Using the variables that we've outlined earlier, let's consider how we would describe the work and play patterns of Ms H:

*Ms H, a 45-year-old woman, has considerable strengths in her patterns of **work and play**. Although trained as a lawyer, she has worked at home, taking care of her two daughters since she had her first child 18 years ago. Although this is **not consonant with her level of training**, it is a mutually agreed upon arrangement with her husband, with which she is **comfortable** and from* *which she derives great **pleasure**. She is very involved with her children, taking them to activities and volunteering at their schools. She has many ways in which she relaxes and **plays**, which also bring her **enjoyment** and help her to **stay healthy**. As a college student, she rowed varsity crew; now she stays physically active by playing tennis several times a week. She is also a member of a book group that meets monthly.*

Variables for describing WORK AND PLAY

Well matched to their developmental level/talents/limitations

Comfortable/satisfying/pleasurable

Adequate for care of self and dependents

Culturally sanctioned

Suggested activity

How would you describe the work/play function of the following people?

Mr A is a 55-year-old man who has been married for 30 years, has two grown sons, and has worked as a sanitation engineer since he was 22 years old. He's proud of the fact that, although he did not graduate from high school, he owns his own home, which he says is the "hub" where his family gathers for dinners on Sundays, Thanksgiving, and Christmas. He and his wife enjoy watching TV, which they do for approximately 2–3 hours each night after dinner. An avid fisherman, he enjoys going to his fishing cabin at least once a month, joined by his best friend and his brother.

Ms B is a 42-year-old woman who is in the 10th year of her PhD program at a prestigious university. She finished her classwork and oral exams 6 years ago and has been writing her thesis ever since. Most of her classmates have graduated, and some even have faculty positions. She is an excellent teacher who has received teaching awards as a graduate student. She is still supported by her elderly parents, who are themselves having difficulty making ends meet. She is unhappy with her academic progress and is unable to move forward with her writing.

Mr C is a 42-year-old lawyer who has been married for 8 years and has two small children. He works in his father's firm, where he struggles to keep up with his fellow associates. He lives beyond his means and constantly feels stressed about money. He was a mediocre student in college, but matriculated at a prestigious law school with the help of his father's friends. Unbeknownst to his wife, he relaxes on weekends by smoking marijuana.

Comment

Mr A has great strengths in both his capacity to work and play. He has steady work that allows him to **care for himself and his family**, with which he is **comfortable**. He takes great enjoyment from being with his family and fishing.

While Ms B's work is **well matched** to her level of training, she is not **comfortable** with her work and it is **not adequate for self care**.

It is likely that Mr C's work is **not well matched** to his level of talent since he is performing at a level that, if not for his family connections, he might not have attained. Although his work **allows him to care for himself and his family**, his anxiety suggests that his work is **not comfortable** for him. He chooses leisure activities that are **not culturally sanctioned**.

Putting it Together – A Description of Problems and Patterns

In this first "Putting It Together" section, we'll illustrate how to DESCRIBE the five areas of function that we reviewed in Part Two. Remember that there are "Putting It Together" sections at the end of Parts Three and Four – as we move through the book, we'll continue to build the formulation. Note that each of these sections will highlight a different clinical case. We'll always start with the presentation, since that's the way you'll first hear the case.

DESCRIBING a person's problems and patterns is the first step toward constructing a formulation. The five areas that we have outlined – **self, relationships, adapting, cognition, and work and play** – give you the scaffolding you need to describe the way a person functions in life.

Let's look at the case of Mr A to see how we might **describe his patterns** in the five areas of function. Here's how he presents at an evaluation:

Presentation

Mr A is a 64-year-old gay man who presents for an evaluation after the death of his mother 4 months ago. Mr A's mother was 90 years old and had dementia. Several years before her death, she had moved to a nursing home in Mr A's town so that she could be near him. In the past few years, Mr A visited her nearly every day. Since his mother's death, Mr A feels "aimless," and "like I'm just drifting." Mr A says, "I know she had a long, good life and I have someone in my life now. I think I should be dealing with this better."

Mr A has been with B, his long-term partner, for 15 years. Mr A and B love each other and are fully devoted to one another but live somewhat separate lives. Mr A works mostly from home doing computer consulting, while B has a busy life as a manager at a bank. B, who is 10 years younger than Mr A, often comes home from work quite late, having had long meetings or work-related dinners. B also travels for work, sometimes for 1–2 weeks at a time. Mr A says that this arrangement has mostly served them well since he prefers to have time alone and B is more social and enjoys the activity. When laws changed allowing same-sex marriage, Mr A and B were quick to have a wedding to which they invited about 50 family members and friends. Mr A says that although people were very supportive of them, the guests were mostly B's friends and he felt somewhat marginal at the event. Nevertheless, he enjoyed himself and was able to manage these feelings. Mr A's mother was present at the wedding. Although Mr A's father, who died 20 years ago, did not approve of his gay life, his mother was more accepting and had become very fond of B.

Since the wedding, Mr A says he has started to feel more lonely. He says his work is slowing down, while B's work seems only to be getting busier. In addition, Mr A says he's started feeling jealous of the time B spends with colleagues and even occasionally feels fearful about B's commitment to him. Mr A says, "B always reassures me ... but I don't know why he thinks I'm so great. He's smarter, more successful, and everyone loves him. Sometimes I think that I just bring him down. I'm lucky that he has wanted to be with me all this time." Mr A says that he is looking forward to retiring but that he's not sure what he'll do with "all that time," adding, "I've never had many outside interests."

DESCRIBE

Problem

Mr A is having trouble adjusting to his mother's death. He feels lonely, aimless, and has some sense that he should be "getting over" his mother's death more quickly.

Patterns

Self

*Mr A's **identity** is not fully established. He identifies himself as a good caretaker (to his mother and to B) and has been reasonably successful in his computer consulting business. However, in the face of retirement, he feels at sea and cannot identify what he likes to do outside of his work. Mr A seems somewhat vulnerable to **self-esteem threats**, particularly in his relationship with B, whom he fears could be cheating on him, although he has no reason to suspect this. Mr A's self-deprecating stance toward B suggests that he may have a less adaptive **internal response to self-esteem threats**.*

Relationships

*Mr A has both strengths and difficulties in this area. His committed 15-year relationship with B is a strength. Lately, however, Mr A has had some difficulty with **trust**, as he struggles with feelings that B could leave him. Difficulty with trust seems be internal for Mr A, as all evidence suggests that B is committed to the relationship. While Mr A must have a good enough **sense of self and other** to have maintained this meaningful relationship, he also has some difficulties in this area. He idealizes B, which has the effect of not allowing him to see B, or himself, in more complex ways. Mr A feels less **secure** in his relationship with B than seems warranted, given the strength and longevity of their commitment to each other. His lack of close friendships confirms that he has trouble in this area. Yet, Mr A is able to tolerate some degree of **intimacy** in that he has stayed with B and also had a very close relationship with his mother. In the area of **mutuality**, Mr A seems to give much more than he takes (in caring for his mother and in his stance toward B).*

Adapting

*In general, Mr A adapts to stress quite well. He **manages his emotions** and does not report difficulty with **stimulus regulation**. He uses a **range** of **defenses**, some of which are more adaptive than others. For example, he rationalizes that B's business trips suit his own need for time to himself. When stressed, he idealizes and projects – his apparently groundless worry that B will leave him illustrates this. His use of altruism (caring for his mother) indicates that he is a caring* person, yet he may use this defense in a less adaptive way in that he has difficulty receiving care and affection from others. He is a fairly **emotional** person who can adapt reasonably well when there are fewer stressors; however, in the face of his mother's death and his upcoming retirement, he has become **less flexible** in his use of defenses. He has no evidence of difficulty with **impulse control**.

Cognition

This is mostly an area of strength for Mr A. His ability to run his own business suggests that he has relatively strong **general cognitive functions**. He seems reasonably intelligent and he has the skills and abilities to manage the work as well as the finances of his business. His thoughts are well organized, and his memory appears intact. His capacity for **self-reflection** is only fair; he understands that he is likely reacting to his mother's death but he is less able to question his jealous feelings about B. This may also indicate some difficulty with **mentalization**, as it is unclear whether he can fully imagine B's perspective (it must be frustrating for B to feel that his love for Mr A is not something Mr A can fully take in). Mr A has no evidence of difficulties with his **judgment**.

Work/play

Mr A has more strengths in his work life than in his play. His work is **consonant with his talents and training** and gives him **satisfaction**. He is able to **support** himself. His worry about his retirement suggests that he is not able to enjoy activities outside of work – in this regard, his capacity for play and relaxation seems limited. All of his work and play seems to be **culturally sanctioned**.

Suggested activity

Now that you've learned about DESCRIBING, try writing a DESCRIBE section for one of your patients. If you're an independent learner, consider sharing it with a supervisor or a peer. If you're a supervisor or a teacher, consider assigning this as a class exercise. It can be instructive to have all of the learners in a class read each other's papers to see how this looks for different patients. You don't have to write about a patient in psychodynamic psychotherapy; this is an important thing to do with all patients so that you can begin to construct psychodynamic formulations in many different clinical situations. Include both problems and patterns. For patterns, use the five headers we've reviewed – self, relationships, adapting, cognition, and work and play – and consider each of the variables in each area. It needn't be long – certainly no more than a page. Remember – don't repeat the history, rather consolidate your thoughts about the problems and patterns.

Part Two References

1. Arikha N. *Passions and Tempers*. HarperCollins: New York, 2007.
2. Freud S. Three essays on the theory of sexuality. In: Strachey J (ed.). *The Standard Edition of the Complete Psychological Works of Sigmund Freud, Volume VII (1901–1905): A Case of Hysteria, Three Essays on Sexuality and Other Works*. Hogarth Press: London, 1905: 123–246.
3. American Psychiatric Association. *Diagnostic and Statistical Manual of Mental Disorders: DSM-IV-R*. American Psychiatric Association: Washington, DC, 2000.
4. Cloninger CR. Biology of personality dimensions. *Current Opinion in Psychiatry* 2000; **13** (6): 611–616.
5. Widiger TA. Five factor model of personality disorder: Integrating science and practice. *Journal of Research in Personality* 2005; **39** (1): 67–83.
6. Kohut H. *The Restoration of the Self*. International Universities Press, Inc.: New York, 1977.
7. Erikson E. *Identity: Youth and Crisis*. W.W. Norton & Co.: New York, 1968.
8. Freud S. On narcissism. In: Strachey J (ed.). *The Standard Edition of the Complete Psychological Works of Sigmund Freud, Volume XIV (1914–1916): On the History of the Psycho-Analytic Movement, Papers on Metapsychology and Other Works*. Hogarth Press: London, 1914: 67–102.
9. Blos P. The function of the ego ideal in adolescence. *Psychoanalytic Study of the Child* 1972; **27**: 93–97.
10. Kohut H, Wolff ES. The disorders of the self and their treatment, an outline. *International Journal of Psychoanalysis* 1978; **59**: 413–414.
11. Reich A. Pathologic forms of self-esteem regulation. *Psychoanalytic Study of the Child XV* 1960; **15**: 215–232.
12. Sandler J, Holder A, Meers D. The ego ideal and the ideal self. *Psychoanalytic Study of the Child* 1963; **18**: 139–158.
13. Kohut H. Thoughts on narcissism and narcissistic rage. *Psychoanalytic Study of the Child* 1972; **27**: 360–400.
14. Neubauer PB. Rivalry, envy, and jealousy. *Psychoanalytic Study of the Child* 1982; **37**: 121–142.
15. Stolorow RD, Harrison AM. The contribution of narcissistic vulnerability to frustration-aggression: A theory and partial research model. *Psychoanalysis and Contemporary Science* 1975; **4**: 145–158.
16. Kernberg OF. Factors in the psychoanalytic treatment of narcissistic personalities. *Journal of the American Psychoanalytic Association* 1970; **18**: 51–85.
17. Cooper A. The narcissistic-masochistic character. In: Glick RA, Meyers DI (eds.). *Masochism: Current Psychoanalytic Perspectives*. Analytic Press: Hillsdale, NJ, 1988: 117–138.
18. MacKinnon RA, Michels R, Buckley P. *The Psychiatric Interview in Clinical Practice*, 2nd edn. American Psychiatric Publishing, Inc.: Arlington, 2006.
19. Fairbairn WRD. Object-relations theory of personality. In: *Psychoanalytic Studies of the Personality*. Tavistock Publications Limited: London, 1952: 152–161.
20. Mitchell SA. *Relational Concepts in Psychoanalysis*. Harvard University Press: Cambridge, MA, 1988.
21. Benedek T. Parenthood as a developmental phase – a contribution to the libido theory. *Journal of the American Psychoanalytic Association* 1959; **7**: 389–417.
22. Erikson E. *Childhood and Society*. Basic Books: New York, 1993.
23. Winnicott DW. The capacity to be alone. *International Journal of Psycho-analysis* 1958; **39**: 411–420.
24. Klein M. Notes on some schizoid mechanism. *International Journal of Psychoanalysis* 1946; **27**: 99–110.

25. Greenberg JR, Mitchell SA. *Object Relations in Psychoanalytic Theory*. Harvard University Press: Cambridge, MA, 1983.
26. Moore BE, Fine BD. *Psychoanalytic Terms and Concepts*. Yale University Press: New Haven, 1990: 133–135.
27. Fonagy P. Thinking about thinking: Some clinical and theoretical considerations. *International Journal of Psychoanalysis* 1991; **72**: 639–656.
28. Fonagy P. *Attachment Theory and Psychoanalysis*. Other Press: New York, 2001.
29. Bowlby J. The nature of the child's tie to his mother. *International Journal of Psychoanalysis* 1958; **39**: 350–373.
30. Mahler MS. On the first three subphases of the separation-individuation process. *International Journal of Psychoanalysis* 1972; **53**: 333–338.
31. Slade A. The development and organization of attachment: Implications for psychoanalysis. *Journal of the American Psychoanalytic Association* 2000; **48**: 1147–1174.
32. Slade A. Attachment theory and research: Implications for the theory and practice of individual psychotherapy with adults. In: Cassidy J, Shaver PR (eds.). *Handbook of Attachment: Theory, Research and Clinical Applications*. Guilford Press: New York, 2008: 762–782.
33. Stern DN. *The Interpersonal World of the Infant*. Basic Books: New York, 1985.
34. Winnicott W. The mother-infant experience of mutuality. In: Winnicott DW, Winnicott C, Shepherd R et al. (eds.). *Psychoanalytic Explorations*. Harvard University Press: Cambridge, MA, 1989: 251–261.
35. Beebe B, Lachman FM. The contribution of mother-infant mutual influence to the origins of self and object representation. *Psychoanalytic Psychology* 1988; **5**: 305–337.
36. Koolhass JM, Martolomucci A, Buwanda B et al. Stress revisited: A critical evaluation of the stress concept. *Neuroscience and Biobehavioral Reviews* 2011; **35**: 1291–1301.
37. Vaillant GE. *Adaptation to Life How the Best and the Brightest Came of Age*, 1st edn. Little, Brown and Co.: Boston, 1977.
38. Bellak L, Goldsmith LA (eds.). *The Broad Scope of Ego Function Assessment*. Wiley: New York, 1984.
39. Bellak L, Meyers B. Ego function assessment and analyzability. *Journal of the American Psychoanalytic Association* 1975; **2**: 413–427.
40. Bellak L. *Ego Function Assessment (EFA): A Manual*. C.P.S., Inc.: Larchmont, 1975.
41. Vaillant GE. *Ego Mechanisms of Defense: A Guide for Clinicians and Researchers*, 1st edn. American Psychiatric Publishing, Inc.: Washington, DC, 1992.
42. Pine F. *Drive, Ego, Object, and Self: A Synthesis for Clinical Work*. Basic Books: New York, 1990.
43. Perry CJ, Beck SM, Constantinide P et al. Studying change in defensive functioning in psychotherapy using the defense mechanism rating scales: Four hypotheses, four cases. In: Levy RA, Ablon SJ (eds.). *The Handbook of Evidence-Based Psychodynamic Psychotherapy*. Humana Press: New York, 2009: 121–153.
44. Freud S. The neuro-psychoses of defense. In: Strachey J (ed.). *The Standard Edition of the Complete Psychological Works of Sigmund Freud, Volume III (1893–1899), Early Psycho-Analytic Publications*. Hogarth Press: London, 1894: 41–61.
45. Vaillant, GE. *Adaptation to Life: How the Best and the Brightest Came of Age*. Little, Brown and Co.: Boston, 1977.
46. Kernberg OF. *Object-Relations Theory and Clinical Psychoanalysis*. Aronson: New York, 1976.
47. Gabbard GO. *Psychodynamic Psychiatry in Clinical Practice*, 4th edn. American Psychiatric Publishing, Inc.: Washington, DC, 2005.
48. Perry C, Bond M. Defensive functioning. In: Oldham J, Skodol AE, Bender DS (eds.). *The American Psychiatric Publishing Textbook of Personality Disorders*. American Psychiatric Publishing, Inc.: Washington, DC, 2005: 523–540.

49. Caligor E, Kernberg OF, Clarkin JF. *Handbook of Dynamic Psychotherapy for Higher Level Personality Pathology*. American Psychiatric Publishing, Inc.: Washington, DC, 2007.

50. Kernberg OF, Selzer MA, Koenigsberg H *et al*. *Psychodynamic Psychotherapy of Borderline Patients*. Basic Books: New York, 1989.

51. Herman JL. *Trauma and Recovery*. Basic Books: New York, 1992.

52. Shapiro D. *Neurotic Styles*. Basic Books: New York, 1973.

53. Descartes R. *Discourse on Method and Meditations on First Philosophy*. Hackett Publishing: Indianapolis, 1998.

54. Cournos F, Lowenthal DA, Cabaniss DL. Clinical evaluation and treatment: A multimodal approach. In: Tasman A, Kay J, Lieberman JA *et al*. (eds.). *Psychiatry*, 3rd edn. Wiley-Blackwell: Oxford, 2008: 525–545.

55. Cabaniss DL, Cherry S, Douglas CJ *et al*. *Psychodynamic Psychotherapy: A Clinical Manual*. Wiley-Blackwell: Oxford, 2011.

56. Spezzano C. Intersubjectivity. In: Gabbard GO, Litowitz BE, Williams P (eds.). *Textbook of Psychoanalysis*, 2nd edn. American Psychiatric Publishing, Inc.: Washington, DC, 2012: 112.

57. Masson JM (ed). *The Complete Letters of Sigmund Freud and Wilhelm Fliess 1887-1904*. Belknap Press: Cambridge, 1985.

58. Brown S. *Play: How it Shapes the Brain, Opens the Imagination, and Invigorates the Soul*. Penguin Books: New York, 2009.

59. Benveniste D. The importance of play in adulthood: A dialogue with Joan Erikson. *The Psychoanalytic Study of the Child* 1998; **53**: 51–64.

60. *Webster's New World Dictionary, 2nd College Edition*. Collins-World: Cleveland, 1970: 1638.

61. Terr L. *Beyond Love and Work: Why Adults Need to Play*. Touchstone: New York, 1999.

62. Vaillant GE. *Aging Well: Surprising Guideposts to a Happier Life from the Landmark Harvard Study of Adult Development*. Little, Brown and Co.: New York, 2002.

63. DeLamater J. Sexual expression in later life: A review and synthesis. *Journal of Sex Research* 2012; **49** (2–3): 125–141.

64. Paluska SA, Schwenk TL. Physical activity and mental health. *Sports Medicine* 2000; **29** (3): 167–180.

PART THREE: Review

Introduction

Key concepts

When we formulate cases psychodynamically, we make hypotheses about how people develop their characteristic ways of thinking, feeling, and behaving.

Thus, once we have a good sense of the problems and patterns, the next step in creating a psychodynamic formulation is to review the developmental history.

The developmental history includes everything that happens during peoples' lives that help shape their dominant patterns of functioning; that is, the way they think about themselves, have relationships with others, adapt to stress, think, and work and play.

When we take a developmental history, we are guided by these principles:

- include nature *and* nurture
- relationships are key
- trauma is critical
- chronology is relevant
- development is lifelong

Although it is important to get a good sense of a person's developmental history early in the treatment, it does not have to be completed in a single interview; on the contrary, our understanding of a patient's development grows for as long as we work with him/her.

Taking a developmental history

Once we have described a person's major problems and patterns, our next step in creating a psychodynamic formulation is to think about when they might have developed. We do this by **reviewing the developmental history** to get a sense of what happened to the person during each phase of his/her life. Taking a developmental history is different from taking other types of histories. For example, when we review the **history of present illness**, we focus on the recent history of the person's most pressing **problems**, and when we review the **past psychiatric history**, we review the lifetime history of the person's psychiatric symptoms and disorders. On the contrary, the developmental history focuses on the things that help shape the **person** – that is, his/her dominant patterns of functioning.

Guiding principles for taking a developmental history

When we take a developmental history, we are guided by the principles discussed in the following:

Include nature *and* nurture

As we reviewed in Chapter 1, people are shaped both by what they bring into the world – their endowment – and by their interactions with their environment. Sometimes when we're thinking about psychodynamics, we think only about environmental influences, particularly the impact of the individual's relationships with others. This is a mistake. An old joke says that psychoanalysts don't consider the role of genetics in development until they have their second child. This speaks to the different ways in which two siblings might interact with the same parents – presumably because of their unique endowments. Thus, as we take a developmental history, we have to ask questions to help us understand the way the person's endowment affected his/her development (see Chapter 9).

Relationships are key

Beyond endowment, we are largely shaped by our relationships and interactions with others. As we discussed in Chapter 5, throughout our lives we have relationships with all kinds of people – family members, friends, colleagues, acquaintances – and each of these relationships is different. Particularly early in our lives, the way we think, feel, and behave actually depends on how we respond to others and how they respond to us. Although this effect is very powerful in our earliest years, it continues throughout our lives, and thus our later relationships can profoundly influence our development as well. Learning about someone's relationships means more than just finding out the names of the key players – it means learning about what those people are/were like and really trying to understand the nature of their relationships with the patient. We will explore early childhood relationships in Chapter 10 and later relationships in Chapters 11 and 12.

Trauma is critical

Compared with the general population, patients who see mental health professionals tend to have a higher rate of adverse early life events, such as physical/sexual abuse and neglect. These events may predispose to difficulties in adulthood, such as depression, anxiety, substance abuse, eating disorders, and borderline personality [1–7]. Thus, trauma can have a major impact on development. However, for a variety of reasons, when we talk to patients, we sometimes shy away from asking about a history of trauma. It can be profoundly distressing and overwhelming to hear about the terrible things that our patients have endured. We may be afraid of upsetting or retraumatizing our patients by inquiring, and sometimes, we don't know what to say.

Nevertheless, it is essential not only to ask whether trauma has occurred at any point in development but also to try to understand the meaning of that trauma to the person. The following are examples of the kinds of questions we might ask to elicit this information:

Can you tell me the story of what happened to you?

What did you feel at the time?

How did you try to understand what was going on at that time? How do you understand it now?

Did you talk to anyone about it when it happened, or anytime after?

Do you see that experience (the trauma) as having lasting effects on you? If so, what?

Do you think that the experience shaped who you are today? If so, how?

Has the experience shaped how you think about other people and how you think about life in general?

When we listen to our patients' histories of trauma, we have to be careful to differentiate between *our* and *their* feelings about what happened. Exclaiming, "Oh my goodness!" in response to a story of trauma might alarm someone who is disconnected from his/her own feelings. On the other hand, making gently empathic remarks such as, "That must have been difficult" can help the patient to know that you were listening and trying to understand.

We also need to make our patients feel as safe as possible in telling their stories and to let them know that we don't have preconceptions about what they're telling us. For example, listening in an interested and empathic but nonjudgmental way as a woman tells you about her experience of being raped may help her to tell the story. Letting patients know that many people have difficulty talking about these things can also be helpful.

Chronology is relevant

In development, *when* things happen is often as important as *what* happens. If the same event happens early in life, it can have a very different impact than if it happens later. Generally, earlier disturbances are more likely to cause pervasive problems than later disturbances. For example, a separation of several months from a primary caregiver at age 1 is likely to cause more global difficulties than a separation of the same length at age 7. We say a problem is **global** if it affects many aspects of a person's functioning, and we say that it is **circumscribed** if it affects fewer functions. If a person cannot form any intimate relationships, for example, his/her difficulty is more global than that of a person who has many close friends but cannot form an intimate romantic relationship.

Once you have a sense of the person's problems and patterns, you will have some idea about how global the issues are. This can help guide you as you explore the developmental history. Because timing of events is so important, we recommend conceptualizing the developmental history chronologically, and we will discuss the phases of development chronologically in Chapters 9–12.

Development is lifelong

To many people, a developmental history is the history of early childhood milestones. While these milestones are clearly relevant, it is important to remember that development continues throughout life, and thus the developmental history must include the later childhood and adult history as well. People grow and change in all sorts of ways in their adult years, for example in psychotherapy! Successes, losses, illnesses, and later relationships all continue to impact the way people think, feel, and behave. We will explore this in Chapter 12.

The evolving history

In the initial evaluation of any patient, you should try to get a sense of the major aspects of the developmental history, including basic information about prenatal exposures, developmental milestones, relationships with primary caregivers, major traumas, patterns of relationships later in life, and the patient's history of education and work. This will help you to construct an initial formulation of the patient that will guide the treatment. However, you cannot learn everything at the beginning. This is not only because it would take a very long time but also because the patient will gradually reveal new aspects of the history as the treatment unfolds. The bottom line is that you need not ask about every aspect of development in your first meetings with the patient BUT you should remember to continue to build your understanding of the patient's developmental history throughout your work together.

How extensive should the developmental history be?

Chapters 9–12 are chock-full of information about development – everything from genetics to issues related to aging. We have included all of this for four reasons:

- to give readers a sense of the range of developmental information that we can learn about our patients
- because mental health professionals learn different amounts about development during their training
- to offer readers a review of this material
- to highlight the aspects of the history that impact the development of unconscious thoughts and feelings.

There is so much information here, though, that you could not possibly learn all of it about every one of your patients. In some clinical situations, such as psychopharmacologic treatments and acute care settings (see Part Five), you may have very little time to get any of this information at all. Whether you are an individual learner or an educator, please use these chapters as a reference. As you read, try to highlight the major points of each developmental phase. Then, when you hear about a difficult period, you can refer back to the related chapter to help you to get more details. The "putting it together" example at the end of Part Three illustrates the type of developmental history that a clinician could write after getting to know a patient quite well. On the other hand, you will find many brief developmental histories in Parts Four and Five. The type of developmental history that you will take in a given clinical situation depends on the amount of time you will have with the patient, as well as the goals of the treatment. But regardless of the clinical situation, you need some sense of the person's developmental journey in order to formulate psychodynamically.

So, let's move on to Chapter 9 and the beginning of development.

9 What We're Born with – Genetics and Prenatal Development

When we think about constructing a psychodynamic formulation, we generally think about how a person's relationships and life history have affected the development of his/her unique problems and patterns. But, more and more, we're learning that people are born with a **unique endowment** that influences the way their relationships and environment affects them. Thus, we have to consider the impact of this endowment when we think about the psychodynamic formulation. We can think of our endowment as everything we bring into the world at birth. It is contributed to by

Psychodynamic Formulation, First Edition. Deborah L. Cabaniss, Sabrina Cherry, Carolyn J. Douglas, Ruth L. Graver, and Anna R. Schwartz.
© 2013 John Wiley & Sons, Ltd. Published 2013 by John Wiley & Sons, Ltd.

- genetics and heredity
- prenatal development, including the mother's physical and emotional health during pregnancy
- peripartum events

This chapter is designed to give you an overview of some of the ways that the prenatal and peripartum periods contribute to adult development so that you can consider ideas about this period in your psychodynamic formulation.

Genetics and heredity

We know that we can inherit physical traits, like height and eye color, but can we inherit the way we think, feel, and behave? These are complicated issues that we have yet to fully understand, but research increasingly suggests that many aspects of our adult problems and patterns have significant hereditary components.

Psychiatric disorders

Twin, adoption, and family studies have long supported a role for heredity in many psychiatric disorders, including mood and anxiety disorders, psychotic illnesses, attention-deficit/hyperactivity disorder (ADHD), and autism [8]. Molecular genetics now provides compelling corroborating evidence for this [9–13]. Although the child of an affected parent will not necessarily develop the parent's disorder, hearing about psychopathology in a parent should alert the clinician to a possible genetic contribution.

Example

Ms A is a 35-year-old woman who presents with depression in the context of a divorce. Although this is the first time that she has sought the help of a mental health provider, Ms A says that she has "always been a sad person." "My family called me Eeyore," she says, "They could never understand why I just couldn't snap out of it." She felt that the one person in the family who really understood her was her maternal grandmother, who herself had severe depression after the birth of each of her children.

Although Ms A's current depression is happening during a divorce, her family and lifetime history of symptoms suggest a genetic predisposition.

Temperament

"I've always been a shy person," says Ms B, "My parents say I hid behind my mother from the time I could walk." Hearing about personal characteristics that people report that they have had for as long as they – or their family members – can remember should make us wonder whether they are describing traits that are related to **temperament**. We can define temperament as the heritable, biologically based patterns of responding and behaving that are

- present from earliest infancy
- consistent across situations
- relatively stable over time [14]

Scientists say that about 50% of variations in temperament may be determined by genetic factors [14, 15]. Several temperamental styles have been shown to be remarkably consistent throughout development. For example, Kagan found that the 4-month-old infants he described as having **inhibited temperament** based on their upset reactions to unfamiliar stimuli were significantly more likely to develop anxiety symptoms by age 7 than infants with **uninhibited temperament** who had responded calmly. These temperamental distinctions have been found to predict behavior in adolescence, as well as MRI findings related to the amygdala in early adulthood [16–18].

In other studies, Thomas *et al.* [19] found that **easy, difficult, and slow-to-warm up** temperaments were remarkably stable over the first 7–8 years of life. **Sensation seeking and avoidance** are other temperamental traits that seem to be heritable and linked to biological markers [20–22]. Finally, neurobiological studies have demonstrated that **impulsive aggressivity** may be rooted in heritable mechanisms for regulating emotions [23–25]. These studies suggest that many traits that have been considered "maladaptive defenses" may be genetically based disordered brain functioning that makes it hard for people to act in healthy ways [26].

Example

Mr C is a 21-year-old man who is referred for therapy by his parents after receiving his third ticket for driving over the speed limit. He tells the therapist that he has always enjoyed the thrill of bombing downhill on his snowboard, bungee jumping, and solo mountain climbing. He's also "less than perfectly safe" in his sexual encounters. He reports that his mother always complained about him, saying things like, "I don't get it! Your sister was such an easy baby! You were climbing out of the crib before you were one!"

The early appearance and consistency of Mr C's sensation-seeking behavior suggests a temperamental origin. Do these early ways of reacting to the world predict our adult personality? Not necessarily. Although some temperamental types are quite stable over time, environmental factors, including early interactions with caregivers as well as other life experiences, can bring about significant changes in temperament. For example, if caregivers gradually expose their infants with inhibited temperament to new situations and challenges, they can help them overcome their propensity to avoid the unfamiliar [27, 28]. Again, although these early ways of reacting to the world do not necessarily predict adult behavior, when a patient describes characteristic patterns of behaving that have been fairly stable since infancy, it's worth considering whether these are temperamental traits.

Prenatal development

Genes aren't the only things that contribute to our endowment. There are 9 long months during which the fetus' brain is affected by a number of other factors, including everything the mother eats, drinks, and, perhaps, feels. The following are among the most common of the myriad influences on fetal brain development:

Maternal habits

Intrauterine exposure to alcohol or cigarette smoke has long been recognized as a risk factor for various cognitive and emotional difficulties in later life [29–32]. Children born to women who **smoke** during pregnancy have been found to have two- to four-fold increased risk of ADHD [31, 33, 34], as well as suspected or definite psychotic symptoms [32].

Prenatal **alcohol** exposure, which is the most common known cause of mental retardation, may cause more subtle but still significant cognitive and learning problems, and, when associated with fetal alcohol syndrome, may cause various psychiatric disorders [35–38].

Example

Ms D is a 42-year-old recently divorced woman who is pregnant with her first child. Her obstetrician referred her because she has been feeling depressed since her divorce and has continued drinking during her pregnancy. Ms D was adopted at birth but recently learned that her biological mother was an alcoholic. Although she was raised in a stable environment with capable, loving, adoptive parents, Ms D has always had trouble paying attention in school. Despite being treated for ADHD, she was a poor student and eventually dropped out in 10th grade.

Although many factors might have influenced the development of Ms D's difficulties, her exposure to alcohol *in utero* must be considered as a potential contributor.

Maternal physical and emotional health

Increasingly, researchers are finding that the physical health of a woman during pregnancy may affect her child's later problems and patterns. Viral and parasitic illnesses, as well as maternal malnutrition in the pregnant mother, have been linked to the later development of various cognitive and emotional difficulties in adulthood [39–48, 60]. Although it is likely that autism is caused by multiple factors, congenital viral infections may play a role [40, 41]. High rates of anxiety disorders, ADHD, conduct disorder, and oppositional defiant disorder have been described in children and adolescents with prenatally acquired HIV [49].

We are used to thinking about the way the emotional health of a person's parents affects his/her development, but we're learning that we have to include the mother's emotional health *during* pregnancy as well. Recent studies suggest that the offspring of mothers with high levels of anxiety and stress during pregnancy have an elevated risk of a variety of psychiatric conditions including ADHD, anxiety, depression, autism, and schizophrenia [50–56]. Although the reason for this is not fully understood, high levels of stress hormones are likely to affect placental blood flow and fetal brain development [57, 58]. Poor nutrition in these women may also play a role [60]. Prenatal depression and anxiety in the mother have also been associated with premature labor and low birth weights that carry their own psychiatric morbidity [59].

Example

Ms E is a 28-year-old married woman who feels demoralized and inadequate about her difficulty staying focused and organized at work. She says, "I can't get reports in on time and I get totally overwhelmed if I have to multitask." She reports that in grade school, her teachers said she was "spacey" and that she had trouble staying in her seat. Although she is unaware of any family history of psychiatric illness, Ms E recalls being told that her mother was weepy and irritable during her pregnancy, couldn't eat because of her "nervous stomach," and spent a lot of time in bed.

Although Ms E's difficulties could have been affected by myriad factors, her mother's depression during pregnancy may have been a contributor.

Prematurity and peripartum brain injury

Finally, we have to remember that the events of a person's birth can also affect his/her development. Prematurity and low birth weight increase the risk for difficulties ranging from cerebral palsy, autism, and mental retardation to ADHD, tic disorder, and OCD (obsessive-compulsive disorder) [61–67]. Brain trauma resulting from hypoxia at the time of birth, the mechanical trauma of the birth process itself, or obstetric complications may also play a role in the development of later psychopathology [68–72].

Example

Mr F presents to the clinic saying that he feels "nervous all the time" and has to "do things" to calm down, like tapping a special place on his bedroom wall eight times before bed, or retrieving the New York Times from the garbage every day "to make sure the word 'God' isn't on the front page." He says that he thinks that he has had some of these symptoms since elementary school. He thinks that his parents overlooked many of these problems because "they were just so glad that I was alive – I was a preemie and weighed about four pounds when I was born."

Given the history of prematurity, it is worth considering whether peripartum events may have been a factor in the development of Mr F's current difficulties.

Nature and nurture – a two-way street

Although the exact origins of our later cognitive and emotional difficulties are not known, research suggests that they are caused by some combination of "nature" and "nurture" – complex, mutually influencing interactions between variations in multiple genes and the environment. These are often called **gene by environment interactions** [73]. It has long been recognized that our endowment can influence the quality of our early experiences with caregivers and may in turn be modified by these relationships and other environmental factors. For example, a baby who startles easily, cries often, and is difficult to soothe may overwhelm the already limited reserves of an insecure and depressed mother who then withdraws from the child, further exacerbating the baby's distress. The quality of early parental care can even modify the expression of genes that regulate the developing infant's behavioral and neuroendocrine responses to stress [74, 75].

Resilience

It's not only our susceptibility to later difficulties that may be related to genetics and prenatal development – researchers are now finding that our capacity for **resilience** may also be hereditary. Differences in the gene that codes for a protein that regulates serotonin movement in synapses (the serotonin transporter, which is the target of many antidepressants) may explain why only certain people develop serious depression after stressful life experiences [76–78], while differences in genes that regulate the metabolism of neurotransmitters may explain why some teenagers who use cannabis develop psychotic illnesses when adults and others do not [79]. Genetic differences of this nature may also affect an individual's response to early childhood maltreatment and trauma [80–85].

Example

Ms G, an 18-year-old college freshman, presented to the campus mental health center complaining of mild anxiety during her first set of exams. She says that coming to college was a "big thing" for her because none of her siblings have been able to graduate from high school. "My family is a mess – my older brother is in jail, and my father has a real problem with drugs. I don't know why, but somehow I just got the 'strong' gene." She does well after a few sessions and is able to complete the semester, and, ultimately, college.

Adult problems and patterns that suggest a genetic or prenatal origin

Several types of adult problems and patterns suggest a genetic or prenatal origin. A few are discussed in the following sections.

Psychiatric disorders, particularly if they begin in childhood and/or are associated with a family history

Example

Mr H is a 52-year-old divorced computer programmer who seeks help for "social isolation." He reports that he used to drive his wife crazy with his constant lectures on esoteric topics of interest only to him and had few friends outside of work. As a boy, he was considered exceptionally smart but "quirky," "couldn't connect" with most of his classmates, and was teased mercilessly on the playground when he'd approach kids and say, "Seven times seven is equal to 49." Mr H adds, "My mother is like me. We even have the same balanced translocation on chromosome 16."

Mr H's lifelong lack of social skills, trouble with social communication, rigid preoccupation with certain topics, and family history of similar difficulties in his mother suggest that his social isolation may be related to a genetically based autism spectrum disorder.

Stable temperamental traits, such as inhibition, sensation seeking or avoidance, and impulsive aggression, also beginning in childhood

Example

Ms I is a 24-year-old recent college graduate who seeks help for "interview phobia." She was recently turned down for a number of positions for which she felt "way overqualified" because she "froze up" at the interviews. Ms I remembers she was always timid and quiet. Her mother told her that as an infant she would cry if she were placed on the rug in an unfamiliar place and that as a two-year-old baby she sobbed whenever someone she didn't know came to the door.

Ms I's "interview phobia" may be one manifestation of a lifelong pattern of temperamental inhibition.

Cognitive and/or behavioral problems with a history of prenatal exposure

Example

Mr J is a 25-year-old man who presents because he is having difficulty at work. "I sort of faked it through school, but now that it's about my job I just can't make all these careless mistakes anymore." He says that he has had significant academic and behavioral problems since kindergarten and that at one point he was diagnosed as having ADHD. At one point during the interview, he pulls out a pack of cigarettes and asks, "Do you mind? I know ... it's a horrible habit, but I've been smoking two packs a day since high school. I was raised in a cloud of smoke – my mother was completely addicted. She died last year of lung cancer."

Mr J's history of ADHD may be related to other risk factors but his likely prenatal exposure to cigarette smoke may have been a contributor.

Taking a developmental history of the prenatal phase

How do you take a developmental history of the time before the person was born? In the treatment of a child, the parents come in to give the history, but in the treatment of adults, we generally have to rely on what they know.

Family history of psychiatric disorders and temperamental traits

Note that this should include asking about the extended family – patients usually tell us only about their nuclear family.

> *Does anyone in the family have a history of mood, anxiety, or psychotic disorder?*
>
> *Was anyone in the extended family ever hospitalized for a psychiatric problem?*
>
> *Did anyone in the extended family ever commit or attempt suicide?*
>
> *Does/did anyone in the family ever use substances?*

If the person seems to have a particular temperament, such as an inhibited or sensation-seeking temperament, you can ask

> *Does anyone else in the family have those traits?*
>
> *Do your family members think that you remind them of another family member?*

Prematurity and birth

> *Were you born prematurely? If so, at how many weeks? Were you in an incubator? For how long? Do you know if your mother had any illnesses during her pregnancy with you?*
>
> *Did you have any surgeries immediately following birth? Do you know what they were for?*
>
> *Do you have any medical problems that you've had since you were born?*
>
> *Do any genetic disorders run in your family?*

Maternal habits and health

Even if your adult patients do not know if they had any toxic exposures while they were *in utero*, asking about maternal habits can give you a sense of whether this might have been a possibility.

> *Did your mother smoke, drink alcohol, or use drugs when you were little? What about now?*
>
> *Is there a possibility that your mother was not eating well or that she was ill when she was pregnant with you?*
>
> *Have you ever heard that your mother might have been depressed or under a lot of stress when she was pregnant with you? What were the circumstances?*

Taking a developmental history from adults who do not know their biological parents

In the era of assisted reproduction, more and more patients will not know their biological parents. This has generally been true of adoptees, but now sperm and egg donation are increasingly common, as is the use of a surrogate to carry a pregnancy. Some people may have some information about a donor's genetic background, or the conditions of the surrogate's pregnancy, but many will not. Some may have information about one parent but not the other. Nevertheless, it is always important to find out the conditions of the patient's birth. Questions like the following can help:

Did your biological parents raise you?

If not, can you tell me more about how that came about?

In Chapter 10, we move from nature to nurture as we consider the person's earliest years, focusing on the way in which relationships shape subsequent development and adult relationships.

Suggested activity

In the following example, try to weigh the likely contribution of genetics and/or prenatal development to the patient's presenting problems and patterns:

Example

Mr A is a 32-year-old man who presents with new onset of panic attacks. He tells you that he was the product of a surrogate pregnancy using a donor egg and his father's sperm. The surrogate did not smoke or drink during pregnancy and maintained excellent nutrition throughout. According to his mother, there were no problems during the surrogate pregnancy, labor, and delivery. However, his mother said, "Your father was a wreck throughout the whole thing! He couldn't believe that we were going to trust the pregnancy to someone else. He was sure that something would go wrong. He didn't sleep for months." There is no known history of psychiatric illness in his father's family.

Comment

There is no known family history of psychiatric illness in Mr A's paternal relatives and no known problems in prenatal development or delivery that might have increased Mr A's risk for developing an anxiety disorder in adulthood. However, Mr A's father may have symptoms of anxiety, and thus, it is possible that Mr A's susceptibility to an anxiety disorder may have been inherited. It is also possible that emotional difficulties were not adequately screened for in the egg donor – this is very difficult to rule out in this situation.

10 The Earliest Years

Key concepts

During the earliest years (age 0–3), children develop fundamental abilities that underlie the way they will perceive themselves and interact with the environment later in life. These include the capacity to

- trust other people
- form secure attachments
- develop and maintain a stable sense of themselves and others
- understand and regulate emotions
- develop language and other cognitive skills

The development of these capacities is strongly influenced by the early relationships that children have with their primary caregivers.

Adult problems and patterns that suggest origins in this period tend to be global and include difficulties with

- self-esteem management and maintaining a stable sense of self
- trusting others and maintaining stable relationships with others
- self-regulation

Taking a developmental history of the earliest years involves learning about the

- environment into which the child was born
- characteristics of the primary caregivers
- quality of early relationships with primary caregivers
- history of separations and trauma

Psychodynamic Formulation, First Edition. Deborah L. Cabaniss, Sabrina Cherry, Carolyn J. Douglas, Ruth L. Graver, and Anna R. Schwartz.
© 2013 John Wiley & Sons, Ltd. Published 2013 by John Wiley & Sons, Ltd.

When you build a house, the first thing you have to do is to lay a good foundation. It needs to be strong, but it also needs to be flexible enough to withstand future blows. The same is true for a developing person, and the years between birth and about 3 years are the time to lay this internal **foundation**. These are the **earliest years**, and they are the time when children are learning to trust and form secure attachments, establishing a stable sense of themselves and others, developing the capacity to know and regulate their own feelings and internal states, and gaining essential cognitive abilities.

Connecting to the primary caregiver

All of this development happens in the context of the child's earliest relationships. Many investigators have speculated that infants are preprogrammed to form relationships, since their survival – both physical and emotional – depends on it [86–88]. For babies, early tactile stimulation – simply being held – can be literally a matter of life and death [88–92]. A lack of early tactile stimulation and physical proximity to the primary caregiver has been found to cause multiple problems, including delays in physical growth and neurobehavioral development [93, 94], depressed levels of stress hormones [90, 91, 95, 96], weakened immune function, [96, 97], and even death [98, 99]. Lack of touch in infancy has also been linked to behavioral problems later in life, including aggressiveness, violent behavior, substance abuse, and depression [100–105].

During the first several years of life, babies must form at least one reliable, consistent, nurturing relationship in which they feel unconditionally loved and completely cared for. This relationship can be with the mother, but it can also be with another person – for the purposes of this discussion, let's call that person the **primary caregiver**. Because this is a one-on-one relationship, it is often called a **dyadic relationship**.

Children who establish a solid dyadic relationship are fortunate indeed – they now have an internal foundation that will serve them well for the rest of their lives. They generally feel that they are capable of being loved, that people will take care of them, that other people understand them, and that their anger will not destroy their loved ones. Conversely, children who do not establish a solid dyadic relationship are likely to have global difficulties in one or more of these areas.

"Good enough" parenting

The dyadic relationship does not have to be perfect – it has to be what Winnicott called "good enough." The "good enough" caretaker is the "ordinary devoted mother ... in her ordinary loving care of her own baby" [102]. Good enough parenting insures that children are generally cared for and loved without abuse or neglect. With good enough parenting, children should be able to develop at least a nascent capacity for all of the things we discuss in this chapter [102].

What develops during the earliest years?

Learning to trust

Once there is a connection, the child can begin to develop **trust**. Trust is vital for forming relationships. Without trust, people experience themselves as essentially alone and unable to rely on others. Mutuality and intimacy, which are predicated on the capacity for dependency, are also impossible without trust (see Chapter 5). The ability to trust others is formed in the infant's earliest years and has its roots in the primary dyadic relationship. When an infant's primary caretaker is reliably available and appropriately responsive to the baby's needs, the growing child develops **basic trust** – the core positive expectation that one's physical and emotional needs will be met and that other people can be depended on to provide comfort and safety [106, 107]. Conversely, if a child's early experience is one in which physical and emotional needs are supplied inconsistently or if the child is constantly frustrated, he/she may develop a deep-seated conviction that the world is not a safe place and that other people cannot be relied on.

Example

Ms A is a 42-year-old woman who seeks psychotherapy to help her to "finally commit" to her boyfriend of 10 years. She says that although she wants to get married, she worries that he will leave her. Consequently, she checks his cell phone texts every night and insists on having the password to his e-mail account. She also says that she has few friends and is considered a "loner" at work, "Ultimately, I'm the only one who will really take care of me." Ms A reports that she spent the first 4 years of her life in an orphanage before being adopted by her "terrific" parents.

Although Ms A feels that she had good parenting after age 4, it is possible that lack of a solid dyadic relationship during her earliest years has made it difficult for her to trust others as an adult. When adults have global problems with trusting others, it is important to consider that they may have had difficulties during this phase of development.

Forming secure attachments

The capacity to form **secure attachments** also has its origins in the primary dyadic relationship. **Attachment** is the deep and enduring emotional bond that connects one person to a special other across time and space (see Chapters 5 and 18) [88]. Based on the work done by psychologist Mary Ainsworth, we generally believe that children develop a particular **attachment style** by about age 1. Ainsworth created an experiment called the **strange situation** in which she observed the way in which 1-year-old children reacted to being briefly left by and then reunited with their mothers. After observing hundreds of American children in this experimental situation, Ainsworth outlined four distinct styles of attachment [89]:

1. **Secure** – In this style, shown by about 50% of American children, the child cries and protests initially when the mother leaves the room, then quickly settles down. When she returns, the child greets her with pleasure, is easily consoled if still upset, and then goes back to playing.

2. **Insecure** – There are three subtypes of insecure attachment:
   (a) **Insecure-avoidant** – In this style, shown by about 25% of American children, the child seems not to notice and does not protest when the mother leaves the room. When she returns, the child may ignore her and not approach her at all.
   (b) **Insecure-ambivalent** – The child reacts with exaggerated crying and protests to the mother's departure and remains in distress while she is gone, but on her return, the child arches away from her if held, seems angry, and is not easily comforted. About 10–15% of American children show this pattern of attachment.
   (c) **Insecure-disorganized** – About 10–15% of American infants protest when their mothers leave, but behave oddly when they return. For example, they may freeze in the middle of approaching the mother, walk backwards, or sit, rock, and stare into space.

The caregivers of securely attached infants respond accurately, appropriately, and sensitively to their baby's crying and feeding signals [108–111]. In contrast, caregivers of insecurely attached children tend to be inconsistent, unresponsive, or rejecting, and seem far less able to conceive of and respond sensitively to their infant's mental state. Not surprisingly, these caregivers tend to be under greater social stress (less help at home, more children, financial problems, or a disruptive partner), have more mental illness, and describe more adverse attachment experiences in their own childhood [111–114]. While these environmental influences are key in shaping attachments, it is also important to recognize that inherited genetic factors may also play a role [115].

Failure to form secure attachments can have significant effects on subsequent development and adult relationships. For example, children previously classified as avoidant are likely to be less independent than securely attached children at age 4, and those who were classified as disorganized are likely to have aggressive, dissociative tendencies in later childhood and chaotic, tumultuous relationships in adulthood [112, 116, 117].

Example

Mr B is a 28-year-old man who presents for "problems with relationships." He says that he hates being alone, but also can't live with anyone. Raised by a series of nannies, he says that his parents were constantly "away on business." At a sleepaway camp for the first time at age 8, Mr B was desperately homesick and begged his parents to pick him up. They were critical of his inability to "tough it out," but ultimately were convinced by the camp director to come to get him. When they got there, he spent the whole time alone in a canoe in the middle of the lake. They finally left.

Mr B, who presents with attachment difficulties in his adult relationships, most likely had an insecure (avoidant) attachment pattern as a child as the result of his parents' perennial unavailability.

Bowlby [118], an early investigator of attachment, is famous for having asserted that early attachment experiences influence later social functioning "from the cradle to the grave." Changes in a person's pattern of relating to others can clearly occur, for the better as well as for the worse. For example, social stressors or negative life events in early childhood, such as illness, death of a parent, or divorce, can change attachment patterns from secure to insecure [119]. Still, in the balance, research suggests that early interpersonal experiences at least "set the stage" for adult relationship patterns [120, 121], and greater attachment security in infancy does seem to lead to better social functioning in adulthood [120, 122].

Developing a sense of others

Infants also use their experiences with their primary caregivers to consolidate their feelings and fantasies about other people. With basically caring and consistent parenting – as well as maturation of the prefrontal cortex – children begin to create internal images of the primary caregiver that help them to realize that when caregivers are out of sight, it's because they have a separate permanent existence. This capacity is called **object permanence** [123].

But even when children know that their primary caregivers won't disappear, they still have rudimentary ideas about other people. For example, they still do not necessarily know that someone can have both good *and* bad qualities. This is true of both themselves and others. If the child feels good, the caregiver is good; if the child feels bad, the caregiver is bad. By about age 2 or 3, however, the image of the primary caregiver becomes stable and enduring and can be maintained even when the child's needs are not being met – this allows children to understand that people can have both good and bad qualities [124]. This capacity, referred to as **object constancy** [125], can only develop if the experience of the primary caregiver is predominantly positive. If it isn't, for example, in the case of abuse or neglect, children continue to separate bad from good in order to protect positive feelings about their caregivers [126]. This interrupts the child's capacity to develop a more nuanced and three-dimensional view of both the self and others.

During this time, infants also develop the ability to **mentalize**, that is, to appreciate that other people can have beliefs, feelings, desires, and motivations that are different from their own (see Chapters 5 and 7) [127–131]. Sensitive caregivers help to develop mentalization in their children by observing their children's internal states closely and treating them as having separate minds – even before they understand this themselves [130]. This helps them to appreciate their own internal experience, and, in later childhood, helps them to understand that other people have their own thoughts and feelings. Thus, caregivers who do not do this can hinder the development of their children's capacity for **empathy**:

Example

Ms C is a 29-year-old married woman who presents for help in "straightening out my husband."
Asked to describe him, she rolls her eyes and says, "I've been miserable from day one. He's at the

office until all hours because he wants to torture me, then he disappears on weekends to play golf. I've told him over and over I can't stand the game!" Asked about her family background, Ms C says she spends as little time as possible with her parents: "My mother never knew how to handle me. I'd have crying jags as a kid and she'd just stand there staring at me, like I was a creature from another planet. She still has no idea who I am. I've told her dozens of times that I'm a vegetarian and every time we have dinner, she wants me to taste her steak."

Although Ms C is describing her *experience* of her early dyadic relationship, the details she provides suggest that her mother did in fact have trouble appreciating and responding to her in an accurate and appropriate way. As an adult, Ms C has similar difficulty seeing things from her husband's perspective, appreciating that he may have his own motivations and feelings, and empathizing with his needs.

Self-experience and self-esteem regulation

Along with being a time to learn about others, this period of childhood is also critical for developing a consistent sense of self, as well as the capacity to regulate self-esteem. When infants have consistent, trust-inspiring experiences with early caregivers, they develop the confidence that they can safely explore the world and face life's challenges. However, if early childhood experiences with caregivers are marked by unpredictability and inconsistency – especially by trauma, neglect, or emotional withdrawal – children are apt to lack a core sense of themselves as being safe, effective, and valued in their interactions with the world.

During these years, children also begin to have a nascent sense of their talents and limitations, which can help them to begin to regulate self-esteem. Parents who appropriately **mirror** their children are excited by what the children are able to do, without overinflating or downplaying it (see Chapter 17) [132–134]. Children who are repeatedly disappointed by their caregivers' lack of empathic feedback or sensitive support often have more extreme problems regulating self-esteem later in life. As adults, they rely excessively on the opinions of others to keep their self-esteem afloat, and they tend to swing back and forth between overly inflated views of their own abilities and deep-seated feelings of inferiority [135, 136].

Example

Mr D is a 53-year-old twice-divorced successful investment counselor who kicks his feet up onto the therapist's desk during the initial evaluation and says, "I'm only here because my girlfriend thinks I'm too moody. What does she know? She's a 27-year-old nightclub hostess." He pauses, watching the therapist's reaction. "I totally lost it when she said she couldn't come to the annual company retreat – I'll look like an idiot!" In describing his background, Mr D tells you his father was a "24/7 workaholic" and his mother was a "professional socialite" who was never home. "They were the kind of parents who'd send the nanny for parent-teacher conferences if they had something better to do."

Deprived of appropriate mirroring, Mr D has an underdeveloped sense of self. He is undone when his girlfriend is unable to be with him, and he needs to devalue the therapist and his girlfriend in order to buoy his fragile sense of himself.

Thinking and self-regulation

The relationship with the caregiver helps the infant to develop many other capacities, including cognitive and self-regulatory functions.

Learning to regulate emotions

Although infants experience feelings from birth, they do not know what those feelings are or how to regulate them [134, 137, 138]. Through their interactions with their primary caregivers, they learn both. When infants nonverbally communicate their needs for soothing, feeding, or sleep, this usually evokes a series of unconsciously coordinated and attuned responses from the primary caregivers [132, 133, 139]. This has been referred to as **empathic responsiveness** or **affective attunement**. Imitation of the baby's actions alone is not sufficient. Caregivers must be able to "read" their infants' feeling states from the baby's behavior and then perform some coordinated behavior that "matches" it. For example, if the baby cries, the caregiver might make a gently frowning face. In turn, infants must be able to "read" the caregiver's response as having something to do with their own original feeling experience [134]. This nonverbal communication helps children get to know, organize, and regulate their own internal states without being overwhelmed and is essential for the development of anxiety and affect tolerance [139–141].

Example

Ms E is a 30-year-old woman engaged to be married in 2 weeks. She is worried she will "faint from anxiety" at the altar and asks her therapist, who is a psychiatrist, to prescribe diazepam. She says she has felt easily flooded and overwhelmed by her feelings for as long as she can remember. Asked about her background, she reports how "excruciating" it is to watch family videos of herself as an infant sitting on her mother's lap: "I can almost feel my 'baby self' getting more and more tense but my mother doesn't seem to notice. She looks completely distracted."

Given this information, there is reason to suspect that Ms E's mother did not appropriately help her to recognize and regulate her early feeling states. This may have contributed to her current difficulty with regulating affect.

Thinking

Numerous investigators have shown that the quality of the early dyadic relationship affects various aspects of the growing child's cognitive development during the earliest years. While general cognitive ability does not appear to be affected, language acquisition and the capacity for abstraction are influenced by the security of attachment to caregivers in infancy [131]. At 20 months, securely attached children tend to be faster language learners and have larger vocabularies than insecurely attached children [128, 131].

Adult problems and patterns that suggest origins in the earliest years

Anything that disrupts development during the critical period from birth to age 3 – including insensitive parenting, abuse, neglect, social stress, or negative life events – will tend to have pervasive effects on multiple domains of development and can lead to global problems in adulthood. Here are some examples of adult problems and patterns that might result from disrupted development during this phase:

Difficulties with self-esteem management and maintaining a stable sense of self

Example

Mr F is a 40-year-old married man who comes at the insistence of his wife because of chronic problems of "getting off the mark" with work. Mr F is bright and verbally gifted, but has had a troubled work history because of chronic problems organizing himself and meeting deadlines. He also wants to be "supersmart and original" but fears he is not, and spirals into a "depressed funk" if the results of his efforts are "only" average. Mr F describes having lived in the shadow of his older brother, a highly successful lawyer. Mr F struggled academically and remembers being berated by his father in 1st grade for being a slow reader and "stupid." His mother was "sweet" but chronically depressed and drank heavily throughout his childhood.

Growing up with an emotionally absent mother and a highly critical father, neither of whom provided accurate "mirroring" of his true talents and abilities, Mr F has never developed a stable sense of his own worth and lacks perseverance in solving tasks and pursuing life goals. He is deeply insecure, overly reliant on inflated ideas about his abilities, and dreams of instant success to maintain self-esteem.

Difficulties trusting others and maintaining stable relationships

Example

Mr G is a 50-year-old man still living with his parents, brought in by his fiancée because of severe panic attacks that developed shortly after he proposed marriage. He tells you that his future wife is "the woman I've always been waiting for" and can't understand why he feels so anxious. Although Mr G has dated many women, his mother invariably found fault with all of them because "she thought they were only after our money." While Mr G insists that his relationships with his parents have always been "the most loving," he has few happy memories of childhood and can never recall being hugged by anyone. He was always afraid of "doing the wrong thing" and displeasing his mother: "She had strong opinions about everything. Nobody was ever good enough for her – not even my father."

From a very young age, Mr G's mother instilled in him the sense that the world was a dangerous place and that people – especially women – are not who they seem to be. This has interfered with his ability to separate successfully and to forge appropriate adult relationships with women, and may be an important psychological trigger for his panic attacks.

Difficulties with self-regulation

Example

Ms H is a 30-year-old woman who seeks help because she "goes to pieces" every time her boyfriend leaves town on a business trip. She feels utterly abandoned, becomes frantic, and then angrily demands that her elderly father drive 2 hours in from his country house to stay with her. She has never slept alone – "not for a single night, ever." Ms H's mother died in childbirth and she later learned that her father went through several years of intense grief, depression, and heavy drinking during her infancy, leaving the responsibility for her care to his half-sister who had three children of her own and resented the "imposition."

Ms H's history of early parental loss and inadequate parenting in her earliest years (by both her depressed father and her overwhelmed aunt) has left her unable to tolerate separations and vulnerable to anxiety when abandonments loom. In the absence of a reliable, loving, early caregiver, she seems never to have developed the capacity to evoke a soothing presence to calm herself down, and she makes frantic efforts to avoid being left alone [124].

Taking a developmental history of the earliest years

People don't know and will never be able to tell you what transpired in their first 3 years of life. This is simply the nature of memory. Areas in the brain that mediate language and autobiographical memory are not "online" and fully functioning until 18–36 months of age [142]. After age 3, people have what has been called **declarative** or **explicit** memory for the events they experienced – they can probably remember and tell the story of their first day in kindergarten. But to make informed guesses about events during those first few "missing" years of life, we have only the patient's **procedural** or **implicit** memory to guide us – emotional responses, patterns of behavior, and skills that are nonverbal and that are unconscious in the sense that they can't be retrieved for conscious reflection. Instead of *telling* us about these events, patients *act them out* every day in their interactions with the world and in their relationships with other people, including therapists. This unconscious or procedural memory about "being in relationships" has been called **implicit relational knowing** [143, 144].

As clinicians, how can we put together reasonable hypotheses about our patient's earliest relationships? It turns out there is great consistency between the nonverbal interactions that take place between an infant and a caregiver during the earliest years and the observable behavior of adults in interactions with others, including therapists [142, 144, 145]. We gain valuable clues about the nature of our patients' earliest formative relationships by paying close attention to how they habitually interact with us and make us feel, in addition to listening to how they describe current relationships [142, 145].

Here are some additional guidelines for taking a developmental history of this time period:

Early environment

> *Where did you live after you were born? In what type of dwelling? How did you come to live there? With whom did you live?*
>
> *What were the financial circumstances of the people with whom you lived?*
>
> *Did you live with your biological parents? If not, what were the circumstances? (e.g., adoption, surrogacy, living in an orphanage, or extended family living situation)*
>
> *Were you adopted? If so, at what age? What were the circumstances of the adoption?*
>
> *Do you think that your parents wanted to have a child when you were born?*
>
> *Where are you in the birth order of your family? How do you think this affected your early years?*
>
> *Can you tell me about your earliest memory?*

Qualities of the primary caregivers

Although adults may not actually remember this, they will have heard stories about their caregivers that are important to hear about.

> *Who were your primary caregivers?*
>
> *What were your primary caregivers like? Do you have memories of them during your earliest years? If your primary caregivers were not your biological parents, can you tell me what the circumstances were?*
>
> *Were your primary caregivers generally happy with their lives? Were they stressed in one way or another?*
>
> *Were your primary caregivers emotionally or physically ill during your early childhood? Do you know if they were drinking or using drugs?*
>
> *Do you know what your primary caregivers' relationships with their parents were like?*

Quality of the early relationships with the primary caregivers

> *Do you think that you were loved and well cared for during this period of your life? Do you remember being held and kissed? Being called pet names? Having your scribbles tacked onto the refrigerator?*
>
> *Are there pictures/video of your early family? What do they show?*
>
> *Do you feel that your primary caregivers were happy to have a child?*
>
> *Do you have memories of being soothed when upset? Who usually calmed you?*

History of separations and/or trauma during this time

> *Do you have any memories of especially difficult or upsetting experiences during this time?*
>
> *Were you physically ill and/or hospitalized during this period? If so, was your primary caregiver with you?*
>
> *Was your primary caregiver absent or inconsistently present during this time of your life?*
>
> *Do you have any memory of physical or emotional trauma, or sexual abuse during this time?*

Note that when asking about abuse, particularly during the earliest years, you may get more information if you ask in this way:

> *Did you have any physical or sexual experiences that made you uncomfortable during this time?*

In Chapter 11, we follow what happens as toddlers begin to explore the wider world and broaden their social sphere.

Suggested activity

Consider the following example and think about what problems Mr A might have had during his earliest years:

> *Mr A is a 25-year-old man who presents for therapy because he has been cutting himself at night when he is alone. "I used to do this as a kid but stopped," he says, "but it comes back late at night when I'm not with people." He says that he was fine in college because "there was always someone home," but now that he is in his own apartment he is having difficulty "settling down." "I don't even know what I'm feeling," he says, "It's just a jumble." Mr A reports that he was raised in foster care because his mother was in and out of drug rehabs, and that he never knew his father.*

Comment

Raised in foster care, with one parent only intermittently available, it is likely that Mr A developed an **insecure-disorganized attachment**. This has likely impaired his ability to achieve **object permanence** and **constancy**, and to **regulate his own anxiety and affect**. This is evident in his need to constantly be with people, his inability to understand his own feelings, and his use of self-mutilation to regulate his affects.

11 Middle Childhood

Key concepts

Between the age 3 and 6, children become more aware of relationships between people in their environment. The idea that their primary caregivers have relationships with each other can produce rivalries and jealousies that affect the way children think about themselves and others.

During this period, children continue to develop their

- sense of self, particularly related to their bodies and sexuality
- relationships with others, particularly related to the capacity to tolerate competition and jealousy
- sense of morality

Adult problems and patterns that suggest origins in middle childhood include

- difficulty committing to relationships
- sexual inhibitions
- fear of competition
- inhibited ambition

Taking a developmental history of this period involves asking about the quality of the child's relationships with his/her primary caregivers and siblings, with particular regard to

- the way the caregivers respond to the child's burgeoning sexuality
- jealousy or rivalry among the family members

From two-person relationships to three-person relationships

As we've discussed in Chapter 10, the infant's first order of business is to establish a solid relationship with **one** person. This is what we've called the **dyadic**, or **two-person, relationship**. The establishment of this two-person relationship allows the child to achieve, among other things, the capacity to

Psychodynamic Formulation, First Edition. Deborah L. Cabaniss, Sabrina Cherry, Carolyn J. Douglas, Ruth L. Graver, and Anna R. Schwartz.
© 2013 John Wiley & Sons, Ltd. Published 2013 by John Wiley & Sons, Ltd.

- trust other people
- form secure attachments
- maintain a stable sense of himself/herself and other people

Soon, however, the child with the solid dyadic foundation leaves infancy and becomes a toddling, talking little person. The world is now wider and more expansive than just the distance between the child and the primary caregiver. There are generally now (at least) three people in the child's world – the child, the primary caregiver, AND another caregiver. During the dyadic phase, securely attached children appropriately believe that the primary caregiver is all theirs and is possibly even a part of them, but now they have the recognition that there is *another* person with whom they have to share their all-important caregiver. The way these three people in the **triadic relationship** traverse this new and potentially treacherous terrain is vitally important to the development of the internal world of the growing child.

Three-person relationships

As children grow, their feelings toward the people in their lives become more complex [146]. Beyond attachment, children now wish for love, intimacy, and physical closeness. In addition, they become more aware that the central people in their lives have feelings of love for each other, and so the one-on-one closeness that they felt in the two-person dyadic relationship changes. Their nascent feeling of being excluded increases their need for love, as there is now a rival for their affection. These childhood longings, although different from adult experiences, often include physical feelings that are the precursors to later sexual feelings [146]. Since the child is generally still solidly focused on the nuclear family (usually, but not always, composed of parents and siblings), these feelings land on the caregivers. Freud [147] was the first to suggest that childhood is a time of intense sexual feelings and that these feelings are generally expressed toward the parents. He named this phenomenon after Oedipus, the fictional Theban king who married his mother and killed his father, calling it the **Oedipus complex** [148, 149]. Three-person relationships are seen in many constellations with many people, such as friends or teachers. For most of us, though, family members are the most central people in our lives, and for children, parents/caregivers are primary. Thus, relationships with family members are generally the most formative in psychological development.

Three-person relationships in today's families

Obviously, in today's world, diversity is the norm rather than the exception. While some children are brought up in homes with a father and a mother, others are raised by grandparents, single parents, or two same-sex parents. Yet, whatever the constellation we're talking about, there is a general tendency, at this stage, for children to start thinking of relationships in groups of three. These "threesomes" can shift in terms of *who* they include but the concept remains the same: there is a child, a desired caregiver, and a rival caregiver. While children naturally alternate in their choice of a "desired caregiver," predictable patterns exist, depending on the gender of the child. For children who will later be heterosexual, the desired caregiver is usually an opposite-sex caregiver; in children who later define themselves as homosexual, the desired caregiver is generally a same-sex caregiver [150].

Conflict in the three-person relationship

For children, this developmental stage is challenging. They face new and monumental changes; before this time, they were content with one-on-one relationships with each caregiver and kept these relationships separate in their minds. The awareness of each caregiver's relationship to the other, and the feeling of exclusion that this creates, is new and complex. Children now want the desired caregiver all to themselves but are afraid that the rival caregiver, in reaction to the rejection, could become angry and hurtful. They may struggle with the conflict between wanting to possess the desired caregiver and relinquishing him/her in order to appease the rival; they may **resolve** the conflict by doing a little bit of both. Where there is conflict, there is anxiety, and where there is anxiety, there is defense (see Chapter 15):

$$\text{Conflict} \rightarrow \text{Anxiety} \rightarrow \text{Defense}$$

The major defense that helps children here is **identification** – they identify with the rival caregiver, realizing that they can become like the rival some day and ultimately have their own intimate relationship, just like the rival's. In this case,

$$\text{Conflict} \rightarrow \text{Anxiety} \rightarrow \text{Identification}$$

So, girl or boy, future homosexual or heterosexual, the child who is securely attached to a primary caregiver has just wandered from two-person-relationship bliss into the confusion and potential danger of a three-person relationship. Is it real danger? Does the child really need to fear the jealous rival? Certainly, in some chaotic, violent households, yes, but these would not be the situations in which the child would have successfully traversed the earliest years. When we're talking about families in which the child is securely attached, we're talking mostly about imagined or fantasied dangers, albeit fantasies that can be augmented or diminished by the behaviors of the important adults involved.

Variations on the three-person relationship in childhood

When this developmental phase goes well, the primary caregivers embrace the child's desires and affections in a safe and supportive way. The desired caregiver allows for some, but not too much, special closeness, and the rival caregiver allows the child to demand the desired caregiver's attention, while also setting appropriate limits. Over time (usually months), children regain closeness to the rival caregiver, while perhaps keeping a special place in their hearts for the desired caregiver. This is sometimes called **successfully traversing the Oedipal phase**.

There are, however, a variety of ways in which problems can arise in the three-person relationship. These problems can affect the child's ability to resolve the conflicts of this period, often leading to persisting fantasies that can affect later development. In the examples that follow, consider how these adults' descriptions of their childhood relationships give us clues to how they navigated their three-person relationships.

The desired caregiver can shun the child

Examples

Ms A, a heterosexual 28-year-old woman, tells you that she adored her father when she was little. She has pictures of the two of them cuddled together and she says, "I've never been as happy as I look in that picture." She remembers that when she was around 5 years old, her father lost his job and became depressed. Ms A says he also became increasingly judgmental, especially about anything having to do with her appearance or femininity. Ms A says, "Maybe it was my fault; I was always bothering him and he wasn't well. I probably made things worse."

Ms B, a 50-year-old gay woman, says, "My mother was just so critical of me. She was always trying to get me to be more 'girly.' In fact, I was a super-good student, particularly in science, and she was a scientist! I actually really admired her, but she just pushed me away, again and again."

In the first example, Ms A's father pulls away from her because of his depression. However, because she's afraid that her love and desire was either too much or inappropriate, Ms A blames herself for his withdrawal. In the second example, Ms B's mother may have become critical because of her discomfort with Ms B's sexuality.

The desired caregiver can be overly receptive to the child

Examples

Mr C, a 25-year-old gay man, tells you that his father was overly focused on his attractiveness and masculinity, particularly in sports. He says, "From the time I was very little, my father was grooming me to be a star athlete. He would come with me to all the practices. He was just too involved! It made me uncomfortable, the way he would brag about me to all his friends, and never mention my sister."

Mr D, a heterosexual 40-year-old man, says that his mother and father did not get along well when he was growing up. While he was unaware of his father's affairs when he was young, he now looks back and says, "I think my mother had a hard time with my growing up. She would snuggle with me at bedtime for years and it got really uncomfortable. It was like she needed male affection and she came to me for it."

While potentially exciting, getting too close to the desired caregiver is generally overstimulating and frightening. The child in this situation is sometimes referred to as an **Oedipal victor** [151]. This can be a particular problem in single-parent households where there is no rival. While longed for in fantasy, the relationship with the desired caregiver feels incestuous, and when it gets too close, it produces anxiety in the child. Plus, the closer the relationship with the desired caregiver gets in reality, the more the child fears the rival's wrath.

The rival is too frightening or rejecting

Examples

Mr E, a 30-year-old heterosexual man, reports that he remembers that, at about age 4, he showed off his bicep to his father, who said, "you call that a muscle?"

Ms F, a 38-year-old heterosexual woman brought up by her grandmother, remembers that her grandmother punished her for trying on her high heels, saying, "they're not for little girls."

In order to resolve the conflicts of this period, the child has to be able to identify with the rival. But in situations in which the danger from the rival feels too real, or in which the rival discourages identification or even mocks or belittles the child's attempt to be like him/her, this is difficult if not impossible. A rageful or envious rival makes identification terrifying and makes attachment to the desired caregiver too dangerous. Mr E's father makes his son's fantasy of ever being like the giant father an impossible dream. Ms F's grandmother makes her granddaughter feel ridiculous for trying to be a "grown-up lady." The shame produced by these rejections makes the attempt to identify dangerous, and it is often repressed as well.

Difficulties in the three-person relationship may lead to repression of sexuality

All of these situations can lead to repression of the following fantasies that are characteristic of this period:

I want to have the desired caregiver all to myself.
My wish to have the desired caregiver all to myself is dangerous.
I want to be like the rival so that I can have my own love relationship someday.

These repressed fantasies then lay buried while children grow up, only to be activated later when they reach the age when they can have their own intimate relationships. This is called **deferred action** [152] – fantasies that are repressed in childhood come into play later in life, and may lead to **symptoms**. They can also lead to the formation of characteristic problems, patterns, and defenses. The repressed fantasies that result from all the feelings and conflicts having to do with three-person relationships are often referred to in shorthand as "Oedipal fantasies or conflicts" [153].

What develops during middle childhood?

As children increase their awareness of themselves and their world during middle childhood, they develop a more sophisticated sense of who they are and how they relate to others. If things have gone well in the earliest years, they enter this period with a nascent sense of self and the capacity to have relationships with others based on secure attachments. But now their growing bodies and minds allow them to develop these capacities in new ways.

Self-perception and self-esteem regulation

During middle childhood, children continue to develop their sense of self. This is fueled by many factors. Some of this comes from new thoughts and feelings about their bodies. Most children consolidate control of their bowel and bladder function during these years, giving them newfound mastery over their bodies and a growing sense of independence. Awareness of gender comes to the fore as children become curious about each other's bodies, as well as their own [146]. Consolidating one's gender identity means coming to terms with what one has and what one doesn't have – this helps not only to solidify one's sense of self but also to differentiate reality from fantasy. Once again, relationships are key to this developmental process – children who feel good about their bodies and their sense of maleness or femaleness base much of this on the way their primary caregivers respond to them. As in the previous examples, the girl who wants to try mommy's lipstick but is told "That's not for babies," may feel insecure about her femininity, while the boy whose father says, "You are getting so strong!" is likely to feel good about his developing male body.

Relationships with others

In middle childhood, children develop the capacity to think about people as having relationships with each other as well as relationships with them. This allows them to feel like part of a family, and even a community (e.g., a day care center or nursery school). While this can enrich their sense of security, it can also lead to jealousies and rivalries as they struggle between wanting someone all for themselves and being able to share that person with others. Learning to tolerate jealousy and competition is an important developmental goal of this phase.

Some of that development can occur in the context of relationships with **siblings**. Siblings can be companions and competitors, playmates and roommates, helpers and hinderers. The presence of siblings means that others are vying for the love and attention of the primary caregivers, but it also affords the potential for alternative sources of affection. When a parent is emotionally or physically absent, a sibling may play a major role in the child's three-person relationship. Too often, when we think about the competitive relationships of middle childhood, we forget siblings, but they are crucial to this period and throughout life.

Moral development

Although children begin to recognize right and wrong at a very early age, their sense of morality undergoes tremendous development during middle childhood [146]. In psychodynamic theory, morality is generally thought to be mediated by a part of the mind called the **superego** [153]. We generally think of the superego as consisting of two parts: one that maps to the **conscience** and one that maps to the **ego ideal** (how we like to see ourselves) [153]. One of the ways that children resolve the conflicts of the three-person relationships of middle childhood is by identifying with their caregivers and by internalizing their caregivers' rules and ideals. These become part of the developing superego. The internalization of the caregivers' rules is thought to help children further develop their own internal set of behavioral guidelines. The first set of internalized guidelines is often very strict: children who are aged 3–6 years are often acutely sensitive to rules and sometimes become outraged if rules are violated [154]. This preoccupation with rules is seen as a normal and universal aspect of navigating this period of development.

The role of temperament and psychiatric disorders during middle childhood

The presence of depression and anxiety can exacerbate the potency of repressed middle childhood fantasies. For example, when a situation in adulthood is reminiscent of a frightening middle childhood situation, the associated anxiety will be worse in the person with panic disorder or mild OCD. Similarly, the expectation of rejection in an adult who was shunned by a desired caregiver will be multiplied for the chronically dysthymic person.

Negotiating middle childhood when there have been earlier problems

We have discussed the way a child who has developed trusting, secure relationships negotiates the three-person relationships of middle childhood, but all children enter this phase whether or not they have achieved stability in their two-person relationships. If children do not trust that their caregivers will take care of them and have not formed secure attachments, the relationships of middle childhood may *seem* like three-person relationships but may *actually* be attempts to secure a solid two-person relationship.

Example

Mr G, a 35-year-old man, comes to therapy for help with relationships. His sessions are entirely focused on his relationship with his girlfriend H. He says that H, who is a successful attorney, is not willing to have sex often enough and that she is reluctant to have him spend every night at her apartment. When the therapist asks him for examples, he says, "Well, the other night she said that I had to go home because she had to work on a brief – something due in the morning. But what about my needs? Couldn't she just have sex first – and then do her work?" Mr G reveals that this has been a pattern in his relationships with women – "I want to be around them all the time – and they don't seem to need or want that kind of closeness." Of note, Mr G was raised by a single mother who worked two jobs – including frequent night shifts – to support them.

Although Mr G sounds as if he's talking about the problems inherent in an adult relationship – commitment and sex – the details of the situation suggest earlier problems. For example, he lacks empathy for H, and he seems to crave someone who will take care of him, rather than someone with whom he can have a mutual relationship. The history suggests that Mr G may have had difficulty consolidating a secure dyadic relationship, leading to difficulties with the development of a secure attachment. As an adult, his craving for a dyadic relationship has been translated into the language of an adult relationship, but, at heart, remains a longing for a much earlier type of attachment.

Adult problems and patterns that suggest origins in middle childhood

Adult problems and patterns that suggest origins in middle childhood tend to be more circumscribed than those originating in the earliest years. Recall that more circumscribed problems are ones that affect one part of a function, rather than every aspect of it. Nevertheless, they cause significant pain and suffering. Middle childhood fantasies that are not resolved early in life often come to the fore once people are ready to begin their own sexual and romantic relationships. Here are a few ways that might happen:

Difficulty committing to a relationship

In people with clearly developed capacities for trust, attachment, and self-esteem regulation, difficulties with commitment are often a clue that middle childhood fantasies might be involved.

Example

Mr I, a 28-year-old man, continues to idealize his parents as "the perfect couple." Although he has had many girlfriends, he always breaks up with them just as things are getting serious, worrying that they'll "never live up to what Dad has."

Mr I's continued fantasy that his parents' relationship was perfect, and thus that he can never have what his father has, is impeding his ability to have a committed relationship of his own.

Sexual inhibitions

When children have been overstimulated during middle childhood, potentially appropriate relationship situations in later life may seem too similar to the early three-person situation and feel incestuous. This can lead to sexual inhibitions in both men and women.

Example

Ms J's father, who had adored her as a young child, became much more distant once she began to mature sexually and date as an adolescent. In college, Ms J had crushes on men but pulled away once they became interested.

When Ms J's father pulled away from her in adolescence, she consolidated a fantasy that the feelings she had for her father in middle childhood were somehow wrong. This fantasy is reactivated in adulthood, preventing her from having satisfying relationships later in life.

Fear of competition, particularly with same-sex rivals

When rivalry during the three-person relationship of middle childhood feels too frightening, competition later in life may feel fraught with the same dangers of the earlier situation.

Example

Ms K's father, who had been a college athlete, attended every one of her gymnastics meets, even when this meant that he could not attend events that were important to her mother. One day, while cleaning, Ms K's mother "accidentally" threw away several of her gymnastics trophies. As an adult, Ms K was passed over for a promotion because she neglected to report important accomplishments to her female boss.

In response to her mother's reaction to her close relationship to her father, Ms K developed a fantasy that competition with women was dangerous. This has led her to repress her competitive feelings with women in her adult life.

Inhibited ambition and self-sabotage in the face of success

Again, repressed fantasies of danger can re-emerge later in life in the form of inhibited ambition.

Example

Ms L's mother, who had been a promising academic star, gave up her career in order to have children. While proud of Ms L's success, she subtly criticized her and mocked her dissertation topic as "pretentious." When Ms L was offered the chance to interview for a prestigious faculty position, she began to experience headaches and feared that she had a brain tumor. This prevented her from traveling to the interview and damaged her chances of being offered the position.

As with Ms K, Ms L's experience of her mother as a "dangerous" rival has led to persistent fantasies of competitive retaliation and repression of her ambition.

Taking a developmental history of the middle childhood years

Adults should have at least some memories of the middle childhood period. The history is likely to be a mix of their own memories and stories that they have been told. For children who are raised in a nuclear family, the developmental history of this period should focus on the primary caregivers and siblings; for those raised in other environments, the history will need to be more broad ranging. In addition, you will undoubtedly learn new historical information as the psychotherapy proceeds. Here are some guidelines for reviewing this period:

What was the quality of the relationships with the primary caregivers during this period?

Were there changes in your relationships with your primary caregivers between the early and middle childhood years?

Was there new closeness with a different caregiver (e.g., the father or a babysitter)?

Did your primary caregiver change in any way?

Has the family environment changed in any way?

Was there any concrete change in the environment, such as a change in socioeconomic status or a geographic move?

Were new siblings introduced? Are they older or younger? What was your relationship with them like? What is it like now?

Did grandparents or other new adults (such as stepparents) move into the household?

Was there any trauma during this period?

Were there any illnesses during this period? Major separations from caregivers? Divorce or other type of loss? Physical or sexual abuse?

Beyond the triad

Once in school, the child's world expands exponentially, as bonds with peers take on greater importance. These relationships, and the potential difficulties associated with later childhood, are a subject of Chapter 12.

Suggested activity

Read the following vignettes and think about these questions:

1. What's happening in the three-person relationship?
2. What fantasies from this period might persist into adulthood?
3. What kinds of problems might this lead to in later relationships?

"Abby"

Abby is 6 years old. She is the eldest of two children. Her father is a college professor and her mother is a homemaker who was a social worker. Abby now has a 2-year-old brother who has asthma and who has been quite sick – it was his illness that ultimately led Abby's mother to stop working and to be home full time. He takes medication and requires a good deal of monitoring by Abby's mother. Since the birth of her son, Abby's mother has gained 30 pounds and is intermittently depressed. Abby's mother and father still go to the movies once a week, but they bicker more in front of the children. Abby is smart and cute and loves to go to work with Daddy – she knows all of the secretaries and they put her to work in the department office. Abby has a doll named Baby who, she says, also has asthma. She pretends that she is the doll's nurse and gives him many shots. Abby recently told her kindergarten teacher that her father is the smartest man in the world.

"Billy"

Billy is 5 years old. He is the beloved child of older, very wealthy parents who went through four cycles of in vitro fertilization to have him. As a very young child, his parents doted on him and he was exquisitely cared for – both parents were very involved and nurturing. The family belongs to a club, and the father is an avid golfer. Billy's father always took Billy along in the golf cart, proud of his little boy in his little polo shirt. Billy liked to be with his Dad – he sat in the cart and read books but was not interested in golf. Billy's father, who learned golf from his father, has become disappointed and has started to leave Billy home when he goes to play golf. Now Billy generally spends Saturdays with his mother, going to the grocery store and staying in his room to read.

"Curtis"

Curtis is a very smart 7-year-old boy. He loves people to ask him questions. He adores math and geography and continuously asks his parents to quiz him on his multiplication tables. As he gets older and understands more, the questions need to get harder. His parents are both well-educated people, but his father is mildly underemployed and is frustrated with his position. One night at the dinner table, Curtis's mother asks a quiz question and his father answers first. His father laughs and says, "Good to know you still can't top your old man." Curtis is a bit deflated and soon asks for quiz questions when only his mom is around.

Comment

Overly close relationship to the desired caregiver

In the context of the birth of her brother, who requires a great deal of the mother's care, Abby has developed a particularly close relationship with her father during middle childhood. She idealizes him, but has also identified with her mother. She is not, however, seeing intimacy between her parents. Thus, she may persist in having fantasies about a special closeness with her father that may lead her to feel that she'll never find anyone as wonderful as he is.

Shunned by the rival

Although Billy had a very close relationship with both of his parents in his earliest years, his lack of interest in golf has led his father to reject him. This could affect his ability to identify with his father and could lead Billy to have a persistent fantasy that he is not a strong man, or to feel that he is not able to replicate his father's ability to attract women and to have romantic relationships.

Rival is too dangerous

As with Billy, Curtis had a close relationship with both of his parents, who mirrored his talents. However, as Curtis shows more prowess, his somewhat frustrated father feels increasingly competitive with his intelligent son and mocks him. Curtis thus learns that competition is dangerous and avoids it. If this fantasy persists into adulthood, it could affect both his ambitions and his ability to pursue relationships with others.

12 Later Childhood, Adolescence, and Adulthood

Key concepts

Development continues throughout life; thus, a psychodynamic formulation must include information about later childhood, adolescence, and adulthood.
  During

- later childhood, children need to develop skills and to expand their ability to form relationships outside of the family
- adolescence, teens need to solidify their identity
- young adulthood, people need to learn to build intimate relationships and assume responsibility for themselves in the world
- later adulthood, people need to build meaningful lives for themselves in arenas such as work and family and to sustain the inevitable losses of aging

  Adult patterns and problems that suggest origins in these periods include problems with

- identity (adolescence)
- intimacy (young adulthood)
- maintaining a sense of vitality and meaning (later adulthood)

Development beyond the early years

When we think about case formulation, we often think about the impact of childhood experiences, particularly the relationships of the earliest and middle childhood years. However, development continues throughout life. Patterns are rarely stable until early adulthood, and major changes can occur later in life.

Erik Erikson was a psychoanalyst who thought about development as occurring throughout life. He conceptualized the life cycle as divided into eight phases and specified the key ways in which people need to grow and develop during each phase [155]. Using this way of looking at development, certain kinds of problems that adults present with suggest that difficulties may have in one or more of these phases. We will use many of Erikson's concepts in discussing development beyond the early years.

Psychodynamic Formulation, First Edition. Deborah L. Cabaniss, Sabrina Cherry, Carolyn J. Douglas, Ruth L. Graver, and Anna R. Schwartz.
© 2013 John Wiley & Sons, Ltd. Published 2013 by John Wiley & Sons, Ltd.

Later childhood: 6–12 years

Cognitive development and building ego function

Leaving aside unusual circumstances, for most children between the age 6 and 12, school is the center of their lives. During this time, children must learn **skills** [155, 156]. They also have to learn how to practice those skills – everything from penmanship to arithmetic to violin – in order to improve and grow. They gain hobbies and other interests, learning to use these pastimes to handle anxieties and impulses and to build self-esteem. Skill building is the biggest growth area for the individual during this period. Children who have difficulty with the games and activities of the elementary years will be handicapped once the tidal wave of hormones and other changes hit them in adolescence.

Relationships outside of the family

Forming relationships outside of the family – with both adults and other children – is another major task of this period [157]. Identification with adults in school can have a major effect on development. Nevertheless, parents remain central figures in later childhood, and they are especially needed during times of stress or transition. For the child who has neglectful or abusive parents, a caring mentor, teacher, or coach can have positive, restorative effects; even a best friend can help. Conversely, abusive school relationships, be they with teachers or peers, can impair self-esteem development. A central task of this period is establishing oneself in the world of peers. Peer life blossoms during this time [158], and bullies and cliques can be devastating to the developing child [159].

Changes in the family

As children get older, the probability that their families will change increases. By the time children are school-aged, their parents will usually have been married for a while, and that means that the probability of divorce increases. Changes in parental finances and relocations may also occur as parents experience their own life changes. Siblings may be added to the family, and deaths of relatives may occur. All of these events can affect the developing child. When discussing these events, it is important to ask not only about the child's response but also about the parents' responses, for example, mother's depression after grandpa died or father's worsened drinking after his job loss.

The wider world

No longer cloistered in the family unit, children may first feel the impact of the wider world during this period. For example, they may first feel the impact of cultural issues [160]. Consider children who are bussed into neighborhoods where they are in the minority after spending their early childhood in a more homogeneous community. As children interact more with the world, cultural differences of all sorts become apparent to them. Role expectations may vary from culture to culture – for example, whether girls should excel in school or whether boys can take ballet – and recognition of these differences may affect the children's experiences of themselves in the cultural milieu.

Adult problems and patterns that suggest origins in later childhood

Adults who present with cognitive difficulties, and who are not suffering from dementia, may have had difficulties during later childhood. The person may have had recognized or unrecognized learning disabilities in elementary school, or other problems during later childhood may have interfered with cognitive development. Children who have difficulties during later childhood may struggle academically throughout their lives. They may feel perennially incompetent and have difficulty using intellectual endeavors to bind anxiety. Traumas that occur during this period can impact learning as can the presence of psychiatric disorders. Consider the child with bipolar disorder or ADHD who is trying to consolidate cognitive function in the face of problems with attention or mood regulation. We want to know not only what the child's cognitive development was like but also how the child and the others in his/her life responded to the cognitive development. For a child who is lovingly responded to, a severe learning disability might not adversely affect self-esteem development; for another child with a highly critical parent, getting B's could be a disaster. School function and the expectations of self and others can have a major effect on self-esteem development and may contribute prominently to the development of shame and even some antisocial tendencies (e.g., cheating).

Example

Mr A is a 28-year-old medical student who presents saying that he is overwhelmed by what he has to do on his clinical rotations. He becomes flustered by the sheer number of tasks that he has to perform, is unable to prioritize them, and cannot organize his work. When the therapist takes a history, she finds that he has had this problem since grade school and that he always had tutors to help him. His clinical rotations represent the first time that he has had to do this on his own.

Mr A's difficulty with organizing his work, which began in later childhood, is now giving him difficulty in an adult situation.

Adolescence: 13–18 years

Identity

If age 6–12 is all about acquiring skills, age 13–18 is all about **identity** [155]. School is prominent too, but adolescence is the time when people really begin to figure out who they are. It's a time of wildly fluctuating identifications. For example, one day Jane loves a certain rock star, the next day she hates him; one day Suzy is her best friend, the next day it's Becca. Every day is something new. This is the norm for adolescents. But by the end of adolescence, young people start to have a coherent sense of self that will help them figure out their place in their world. To be able to plan ahead as a young adult, adolescents have to make sense of where they came from. Interest in one's ethnic and religious background increases; adopted children often have interest in their families of origin.

Body changes

For adolescents, the new things happening in the body can be overwhelming. Like the addition of an enzyme, hormones can cause dramatic changes in the developing character. There are many things to consider in a psychodynamic formulation that come to the fore in adolescence. For example, gender issues are usually consolidated much earlier; however, any residual confusion will wreak havoc during this period. Sexual identity may be somewhat fluid for adolescents and experimentation is the norm; however, if differences are not accepted by important others, this can be a devastating time [161]. Masturbation becomes frequent during adolescence, but is prohibited in some cultures and by some religions. Inhibitions and fears about masturbation and sexuality can be particularly painful during adolescence, as the growing individual is often unsure about sexuality and is thus more vulnerable to shame and harsh moral judgments.

Cognitive and emotional difficulties

Adolescence may also be the time when cognitive and emotional difficulties first appear. Early signs of depression often occur and are too frequently ignored or minimized as normal "teen brooding" [162]. Eating disorders and suicidal ideation are common, as are first experiments with substance use [163, 164]. All of these affect the teen's sense of self and self-esteem, as they can affect one's nascent feeling of mastery over one's environment. Consider the adolescent who is just adjusting to the self-esteem blow of not being as smart as an older sibling and who then develops new-onset depression. This person will have to work twice as hard to maintain an already vulnerable sense of self. Good early development helps here, but is not necessarily fully protective against the blows of adolescence. Regressions are common and normal as new experiences and difficulties challenge the developing self – many recover, others do not.

Many factors can disrupt identity consolidation in adolescence. As always, traumas, family strife, and losses have to be considered. A very common source of trouble in this area is substance abuse – drugs and alcohol [165]. Trying to consolidate identity under the influence of substances that alter mood and self-experience is like trying to set Jell-O in a blender. It doesn't happen. The same is true for the influence of other cognitive and emotional difficulties, such as bipolar disorder and panic attacks.

Adult problems and patterns that suggest origins in adolescence

Adults who present without a good sense of identity are likely to have had difficulties during their adolescent years. People who are still "finding themselves" in their 30s and beyond may not have had an adequate chance to experiment with different ways of thinking about themselves and the world or may have gotten lost during that period of experimentation as a result of trauma or cognitive and emotional difficulties.

Example

Ms B, a 43-year-old married, successful lawyer with two teenage children, presents saying that she feels unfulfilled in her life. Although she is not depressed, she says that she is "just going through the motions" at work and dreams of having a different kind of life. She flirts with running off to a writers' colony, or traveling to India to study yoga. She continuously changes her hairstyle and color and is easily bored with her wardrobe. She reports that her mother died when she was 12 years old and she assumed primary responsibility for the care of her 7-year-old brother because her father was an alcoholic. This involved staying with him on nights and weekends, foregoing the social life in which her peers were engaged. She chose to become a lawyer early in order to ensure financial stability for the family.

Forced to assume adult responsibilities early, Ms B was not able to try out different choices in order to consolidate her identity; this need re-emerged later, perhaps as her own children began their teenage experimentation.

Young adulthood: 18–23 years

Intimate relationships and sexuality

Emerging from adolescence with a nascent sense of self, the young adult is ready to share that self with another person [155]. The capacity for love relationships, which is built on many years of relationships with family members and friends, can help the individual to consolidate identity. Even people whose familial relationships have been less than ideal can have their self-esteem positively reenforced by mutually satisfying relationships with lovers and friends during this time. However, if the wounds of earlier life have left the person unable to form intimate relationships, this time can be lonely and full of disappointment.

Sexual difficulties may also become prominent as young adults try to negotiate adult sexuality [155]. Sometimes, this can be the result of repressed unconscious fantasies from middle childhood, which can lead to sexual inhibitions and maladaptive relationships (see Chapter 11). For example, the little girl whose young father adored her may be unable to find a man who is "as good as Daddy was," leading her to destroy many a promising relationship.

Responsibilities in the world

Minors no longer, young adults have newfound freedoms and responsibilities. Many leave home and are challenged to function as adults for the first time. How does their sense of self hold up? Can they self-regulate? Remain organized? Care for themselves? This is a time of tremendous growth and excitement for some, and terror for others. Some write PhD's, whereas others go into debt due to an inability to curb impulses. It can be a time of unlimited possibilities or of depression if ambitions exceed capabilities. Negotiating the discrepancies between ambitions and talents in a realistic way is a key challenge of this period – those who do it well gain focus, while those who do it poorly struggle with fragile self-esteem and despair. Identity consolidation continues during this period, as people choose partners and career paths. The fluid identity that is normal in a 14-year-old is no longer normal in a 24-year-old, and ongoing instability in one's sense of self may be the harbinger of maladaptive patterns.

Cultural factors must also be taken into consideration. What cultural issues do newly minted adults confront? Are they members of a minority? How does that affect their self-esteem development? Are they immigrants or first-generation Americans? Imagine a first-generation young adult in a community of white Americans – will that person feel attractive? Shunned? Excluded? Will he or she be able to find a partner? Maybe "yes" and maybe "no," but this should be investigated. Religious differences can also affect the young adult's ability to form relationships during this period.

Adult problems and patterns that suggest origins in young adulthood

Difficulty assuming responsibility for oneself during young adulthood can leave people overly dependent on their family of origin as they enter their third and fourth decades of life. This can lead to mood and anxiety symptoms as they feel unable to mature alongside their peers.

Example

After college, Mr C had several years of severe depression, during which he moved back into his parents' home. Finally stabilized at age 27, Mr C felt awkward with women and delayed in his career development. He continued to live at home, and ultimately went to work for the family business.

Mr C's difficulties assuming responsibility during young adulthood inhibited his ability to develop an intimate love relationship during this time. This resulted in severe limitations in his capacity for adult relationships with others.

Adulthood: 23 years and beyond

The tasks of adulthood are myriad and diverse. Most, however, involve finding sustained meaning in work and love [155]. Some find meaning in family life, some in career, and some in both – as a psychotherapist, it is important to put personal judgment aside and discover what is important to each individual. For example, one person might be content to be an accomplished artist who has always lived alone, while another might feel chronically unfulfilled despite having a successful career and a healthy family. This can be an exciting time of productivity and procreation, but it can also be a time of disappointment and unfulfilled dreams. Asking not only about what people are doing and with whom they have relationships but also how they feel about "how things turned out" can help you in assessment.

Later adulthood can bring the joys of a life well-lived, or the bitterness of a difficult journey. Older adults may lose many things, including physical and mental capacities, opportunities for productivity, the daily routines of work–life, and loved ones. Although the earliest years are far away, the capacities developed during those years (such as trust, sense of self, and secure attachments) continue to play a role during times of loss, buoying the older adult through difficult waters. Valliant [166] has shown that having good relationships is the best predictor of mental health during the older years – relationships based on trust, attachment, and a healthy sense of self and other.

Example

Dr D, a famous surgeon with an international reputation by age 45, has a serious car accident at age 50 that renders him unable to operate. Despite his academic standing and supportive family, he withdraws into himself and begins abusing alcohol. This alienates his family, and he spends many years in near isolation.

Unable to adapt to the loss of his ability to do his chosen work, Dr D is unable to buoy his self-esteem and plunges into depression and substance use.

Taking a developmental history of these periods

Most adults have clear memories of these periods and should be able to give a clear developmental history. Major memory gaps for this time could indicate a history of trauma, medical illness, or substance abuse. Here are some guidelines for taking a developmental history of these diverse developmental phases:

Later childhood

How was your time in school?

Did you have any learning problems? Were you ever tested for learning disabilities?

Do you remember having friends?

What kinds of activities were you involved in?

Were there any changes in your family during this time?

Do you remember this as a time when you were particularly anxious or depressed?

Did you have any illnesses during this period? Take any medications?

Did you ever get into any serious trouble during this time?

Did anything especially disturbing or traumatic happen?

Although people may not know whether they had a frank psychiatric disorder during these years, they will usually remember their general difficulties. For example, a patient might deny having had ADHD, but may be able to say that he/she had great difficulty in school, was constantly in trouble for not being able to sit still, and could never finish reading a book. Remember, though, that there is about a one-in-three chance that your adult patient had some form of a diagnosable psychiatric disorder dating back to childhood. A history of early cognitive and/or emotional difficulties may shed light on the origins of your patient's current problems. The following types of questions will help you to learn about your adult patient's history of early symptomatology:

When you were growing up, did you ever see a psychiatrist, therapist, or school counselor? If so, for what type of problem?

Were you told that you had a behavioral problem? If so, what type?

Did you have to go to a special school? Do you know what kind of school it was?

As a child, did you ever take medication for a behavioral problem?

Do you remember being very sad or nervous as a child? Do you think that you were like that for a long time? For how long?

Were you ever so sad or nervous that it prevented you from doing things like going to school or playing with friends?

Did you have difficulty in school? If so, what kind of difficulty?

Did teachers tell your parents about any particular problems they noticed in you in school?

Did you tend to get in trouble in school? If so, for what kind of behavior?

Adolescence

How do you remember your teenage years? Do you remember it as a happy time? A stormy time?

What was your relationship like with your parents during this time?

Can you remember when you began to develop physically? Was it around the same time as your peers? If early or late, how did this affect you?

Did you have any new difficulties during this time, like anxiety or depression?

Did you try any substances as a teenager? If yes, was this sporadic, or did you use any substances on a regular basis? Which one(s)?

Did you have a boyfriend or girlfriend during this period?

What kind of sexual experiences did you have during this time?

Were there any changes in your family or living situation during this time?

Any illnesses or traumatic situations?

Young adulthood

How far did you continue in school? Did you attend college or graduate school?

Did you continue to live at home? If not, where did you live? With whom?

What were your aspirations at this point in your life? How did you try to realize them?

How do you remember this time? Fulfilling? Disappointing? Frustrating?

Were you involved with anyone romantically during this period of your life? Sexually? What were these relationship(s) like?

Tell me about your social life during this time. Did you have friends? How close do you feel you were to them? Did you tend to socialize one-on-one or in a group?

Did you begin to support yourself during this period? If so, how? If not, who was supporting you?

If you were working, what type of work did you do? Was this what you wanted to do?

Did you find time for leisure? If so, what did you like to do during this time?

Did you have any particular difficulties during this time, such as anxiety, depression, or substance abuse? Traumatic situations?

Adulthood

Tell me about your work history during your adult life. Are you/have you been satisfied with what you are doing? Have you been able to support yourself (and your family, if applicable)?

Who is in your family? If you have started your own family, when did you do this? How do you find your family life?

How do you spend your leisure time? Is this satisfying to you?

Have you had any medical or psychiatric difficulties in your adult life? Substance abuse?

Are you currently sexually active? Can you tell me about this?

Have you lost any people with whom you were close?

As you look at your life, do you feel that you have been happy with the choices that you have made? Can you tell me more about that?

Remembering the whole life cycle

The above outline is not intended to be comprehensive; rather, it is designed to remind you of the many changes that occur after early childhood development and can affect the way in which the individual regulates self-esteem, has relationship with others, and adapts to stressful situations. New problems emerge, old problems reemerge in new clothing, and new experiences and relationships can breed new traumas as well as the hope of repair. These are all things to think about as you review the development of your adult patients.

Suggested activity

During which period of development might these people have had difficulty?

Ms A is a 48-year-old mother of three. She married her childhood sweetheart and has been very happy as a stay-at-home mother but, as her children have become more independent, she has become bored. She has briefly taken up many hobbies including tennis, needlepoint, yoga, and kickboxing, but she doesn't stick with any of them for long. Recently, she has noticed that she is attracted to her personal trainer. This has felt exciting and frightening, and she is not sure what to do.

Mr B, a 56-year-old man, has worked in the library of a famous museum for 30 years. His coworkers admire him for his encyclopedic knowledge of Etruscan archaeology, but fear his biting sarcasm and are loathe to interact with him. Although he graduated with high honors from a PhD program in art history, he was never able to land a tenure-track position at a college or university. He has never had a relationship and lives in very modest circumstances. "No one is producing anything in academia anymore," he grumbles. "I'm glad that I never got into that rat race."

Comment

Ms A seems to have difficulty with identity and is confused about her attraction to a man other than her husband. It is likely that she was not able to experiment enough as an adolescent, perhaps because of her premature attachment to her future spouse. Although this may not have been a problem while she was busy with small children, her newfound personal time has exposed these developmental difficulties, leaving her bored, listless, and sexually dissatisfied.

Mr B seems to have had difficulty in young adulthood. Although his relationship difficulties may predate this time, his inability to find an academic job after his educational success left him unable to realize his talents and led to bitterness and isolation.

Putting it Together – A Developmental History

Now we're ready to to REVIEW a full developmental history. Let's consider how we might do this for Ms B:

Presentation

Ms B is a 26-year-old single white Catholic Intensive Care Unit (ICU) nurse who presents with mounting depression, anxiety, and passive suicidal thoughts – symptoms she hasn't experienced since her teens. Ms B describes "slipping into a black hole" starting 3 months ago when her mother began calling more frequently, pleading with Ms B to help care for her mentally and physically disabled father. Ms B had been planning to leave her ICU job in a year or two to fulfill a lifelong dream of working in a third-world country, but now feels obligated to stay. She feels increasingly nervous, exhausted, and irritable, but does not have difficulty with sleep or appetite.

Developmental history

Genetics and prenatal development

Ms B is an only child born to initially unmarried parents. She is unaware of any problems with her mother's pregnancy or delivery but assumes her mother drank during the pregnancy since she was hospitalized for depression and alcoholism shortly after Ms B's birth. There is also an extensive history of depression and alcoholism in numerous relatives on her mother's side of the family. Ms B's father has a long history of temper-control issues but never sought psychiatric treatment until he was diagnosed with Parkinson's disease 12 years ago; he is now chronically psychotic on antiparkinsonian medications.

Earliest years (birth to age 3)

Shortly after delivery, Ms B was placed in the care of her maternal grandmother. Ms B presumes that this was because of her mother's hospitalization but is not sure why her father could not care for her. Her grandmother told her she was a healthy, relaxed, "easy" baby who almost never cried and who was generally slow to warm up with other children. She has very warm memories of her early childhood with her grandmother, but few memories of her parents during these years – she was told by her grandmother that they were working hard to save money so they could take care of her again.

Middle childhood relationships (age 3–6)

When Ms B was 4 years old, her parents married and moved with her to a neighboring town where her father joined a private investigation company. He made a good living and the family lived a comfortable middle-class life. However, during Ms B's childhood, her father was volatile, harshly critical, slammed doors, frequently yelled at and struck her mother in front of Ms B, and occasionally slapped or threatened Ms B with a belt. Ms B remembers feeling frightened of her father as a child and hiding in a closet when her parents argued. She remembers her mother as irritable and depressed, especially when she was drinking. When drinking, Ms B's mother told her that she was an "unwanted pregnancy" and that she would have had an abortion if she hadn't been Catholic. This made Ms B feel that she was the reason for her parents' unhappy relationship. The only good memories she has of these years were the occasional weekends and holidays she spent with her grandmother.

Later childhood (age 6–12)

Ms B's parents placed her in an all-girls' Catholic school, starting in kindergarten. She loved the school and says it "saved my life." She remembers being shy and well behaved and having close relationships with the nuns and priests. Although she had few friends, she had one close friend to whose home she went most days after school. In middle school, at the urging of one of the nuns, Ms B started confirmation classes and began going to Mass every Sunday by herself. When her parents refused to be involved, her friend's parents offered to stand in as her sponsors.

Adolescence (age 13–18)

When she was 14 years old, Ms B's parents said they could no longer afford the parish school and placed her in a large co-ed public high school. She missed her friends and the nuns at her old school; her grades slipped and she had thoughts of suicide. She also experimented with anorexia and lost 15 pounds but stopped when no one noticed. In 10th grade, a coach encouraged her to try out for the basketball team and she says that she went from "being invisible to being the star player." She started feeling better about herself and made an effort to eat a healthier diet because she felt she had a "responsibility to the team." She loved sports although her mother told her that it was "unfeminine." She avoided parties, immersed herself in schoolwork and athletics, and excelled at both. During the summer between 11th and 12th grade, Ms B volunteered as a candy striper at a local hospital and "just knew" that she would ultimately pursue a career in the helping professions. In hindsight, she thinks her father's nascent Parkinson's disease may have influenced her decision: "The more disabled he became, the less angry I felt. He went from terrifying to needy and pathetic. I also hated seeing how much my mother seemed to enjoy tormenting him and felt like I had to protect him."

Young adulthood (age 18–23)

When the time came to apply to college, Ms B's mother was preoccupied with her father's health issues and financial worries and informed her that if she wanted to go, she'd have to handle the tuition costs on her own. An excellent student and athlete, Ms B had her pick of elite colleges but, wanting to go as far from home as possible, she chose a modest liberal arts college across the country where she was offered a full scholarship. She devoted herself to schoolwork and sports, and, although she joined a sorority, she tended to shy away from weekend partying and had limited dating experiences. She had a number of short-lived relationships with men who "wouldn't take no for an answer" but none of these lasted more than a year. Ms B was initially a pre-med major but, because of her frequent trips home to help care for her father, she "never had the time to master organic chemistry and physics" and eventually switched to nursing.

Later adulthood (age 23 to present)

Once she began working, Ms B was drawn to intensive care nursing because of the "challenge of the life-and-death moments." She quickly rose through the ranks, taking on leadership and teaching positions in the medical center. In the last few years, she has distanced herself from friends, only dated sporadically, and concentrated on her work, her family, and her cat.

Suggested activity

As you did after DESCRIBE, try to take time now to REVIEW the developmental history of one of your patients. Again, classroom learners will benefit from reading the reviews that their classmates write. As in this example, try using the headers from each developmental phase – prenatal, earliest years, middle childhood, later childhood, adolescence, young adulthood, and adulthood. Even if you think that you have a sense of your patient's developmental history, challenging yourself to review it systematically is likely to help you to learn more about your patient and to identify things about which you might want to ask.

Part Three References

1. Kessler RC, Davis CG, Kendler KS. Childhood adversity and adult psychiatric disorder in the US National Comorbidity Survey. *Psychological Medicine* 1997; **27** (5): 1101–1119.
2. Cohen P, Brown J, Smaile E. Child abuse and neglect and the development of mental disorders in the general population. *Developmental Psychopathology* 2001; **13** (4): 981–999.
3. Lansford JE, Dodge KA, Pettit GS *et al.* A 12-year prospective study of the long-term effects of early child physical maltreatment on psychological, behavioral, and academic problems in adolescence. *Archives of Pediatric Adolescent Medicine* 2002; **156** (8): 824–830.
4. Edwards VJ, Holden GW, Felitti VJ *et al.* Relationship between multiple forms of childhood maltreatment and adult mental health in community respondents: Results from the adverse childhood experiences study. *American Journal of Psychiatry* 2003; **160** (8): 1453–1460.
5. Green JG, McLaughlin KA, Berglund PA *et al.* Childhood adversities and adult psychopathology in the National Comorbidity Survey Replication (NCS-R) I: Associations with first onset of DSM-IV disorders. *Archives of General Psychiatry* 2010; **67** (2): 113–125.
6. Clemmons JC, Walsh K, DiLillo D *et al.* Unique and combined contributions of multiple child abuse types and abuse severity to adult trauma symptomatology. *Child Maltreatment* 2007; **12** (2): 172–181.
7. Van der Kolk BA, Hostetler A, Herron N *et al.* Trauma and the development of borderline personality disorder. *Psychiatric Clinics of North America* 1994; **17** (4): 715–730.
8. Plomin R, Owen MJ, McGuffin P. The genetic basis of complex human behaviors. *Science* 1994; **264**: 1733–1739.
9. Ferreira MAR, O'Donovan MC, Meng YA. Collaborative genome-wide association analysis supports a role for ANK3 and CACNA1C in bipolar disorder. *Nature Genetics* 2008; **40** (9): 1056–1058.
10. Sullivan PF. The psychiatric GWAS consortium: Big science comes to psychiatry. *Neuron* 2010; **68** (2): 182–186.
11. Ripke S, Sanders AR, Kendler KS *et al.* Genome-wide association study identifies five new schizophrenia loci. *Nature Genetics* 2011; **43** (10): 969–976.
12. Sklar P, Ripke S, Scott LJ. Large-scale genome-wide association analysis of bipolar disorder identifies a new susceptibility locus near ODZ4. *Nature Genetics* 2011; **43** (10): 977–983.
13. Kang HJ, Kawasawa YI, Cheng F *et al.* Spatio-temporal transcriptome of the human brain. *Nature* 2011; **478** (7370): 483–489.
14. Rothbart M. *Becoming Who We Are: Temperament and Personality in Development*. Guilford Press: New York, 2011.
15. Bouchard TJ, Lykken DT, McGue M *et al.* Sources of human psychological differences: The Minnesota study of twins reared apart. *Science* 1990; **250** (4978): 223–228.
16. Kagan J, Snidman N, Kahn V *et al.* The preservation of two infant temperaments into adolescence. *Monographs of the Society for Research in Child Development* 2007; **72** (2): 95.
17. Kagan J. *The Temperamental Thread: How Genes, Culture, Time, and Luck Make Us Who We Are*. Dana Press: New York, 2010.
18. Schwartz CE, Wright CI, Shin LM *et al.* Inhibited and uninhibited infants "grown up": Adult amygdalar response to novelty. *Science* 2003; **300**: 1952–1953.
19. Thomas A, Chess S, Birch HG. *Temperament and Behavior Disorders in Children*. New York University Press: New York, 1963.
20. Zuckerman M. *Psychobiology of Personality*. Cambridge University Press: New York, 1991.
21. Zuckerman M. *Sensation Seeking and Risky Behavior*. American Psychological Association: Washington, DC, 2007.

22. Zald DH, Cowan RL, Riccardi P *et al.* Midbrain dopamine receptor availability is inversely associated with novelty-seeking traits in humans. *Journal of Neuroscience* 2008; **28** (53): 14372–14378.

23. Siever, LJ. Neurobiology of aggression and violence. *American Journal of Psychiatry* 2008; **165** (4): 429–442.

24. Frankle WG, Lombardo I, New AS *et al.* Brain serotonin transporters distribution in subjects with impulsive aggressivity: A positron emission study. *American Journal of Psychiatry* 2005; **162** (5): 915–923.

25. Coccaro EF, Siever LJ. Neurobiology. In: Oldham JM, Skodol AE, Bender DS (eds.). *The American Psychiatric Publishing Textbook of Personality Disorders.* American Psychiatric Publishing, Inc.: Washington, DC, 2007: 155–171.

26. Hoermann S, Zupanick CE, Dombeck M. Biological factors related to the development of personality disorders (*Nature*). http://www.mentalhelp.net/poc/center_index.php?id=8&cn=8 (accessed 28 October 2011).

27. Partridge T. Biological and caregiver correlates of behavioral inhibition. *Infant and Child Development* 2003; **12**: 71–87.

28. Cicchetti D, Ganiban J, Baarnett D. Contributions from the study of high-risk populations to understanding the development of emotion regulation. In: Garber J, Dodge KA (eds.). *The Development of Emotion Regulation and Dysregulation.* Cambridge University Press: Cambridge, 1991: 15–48.

29. Nichols P, Chen T. *Minimal Brain Dysfunction: A Prospective Study.* Lawrence Erlbaum: Hillsdale, NJ, 1981.

30. Milberger S, Biederman J, Faranone S *et al.* Is maternal smoking a risk factor for attention deficit hyperactivity disorder in children? *American Journal of Psychiatry* 1996; **153**: 1138–1143.

31. Huizink A, Mulder E. Maternal smoking, drinking or cannabis use during pregnancy and neurobehavioral and cognitive functioning in human offspring. *Neuroscience and Biobehavioral Reviews* 2006; **30** (1): 24–41.

32. Zammit S, Horwood J, Thompson A *et al.* Maternal tobacco, cannabis and alcohol use during pregnancy and risk of adolescent psychotic symptoms in offspring. *The British Journal of Psychiatry* 2009; **195** (4): 294–300.

33. Lindblad F, Hjern A. ADHD after fetal exposure to maternal smoking. *Nicotine & Tobacco Research: Official Journal of the Society for Research on Nicotine and Tobacco* 2010; **12** (4): 408–415.

34. Obel C, Olsen J, Henriksen TB *et al.* Is maternal smoking during pregnancy a risk factor for hyperkinetic disorder? Findings from a sibling design. *International Journal of Epidemiology* 2011; **40** (2): 338–345.

35. Streissguth A, Bookstein F, Barr H *et al.* Risk factors for adverse life outcomes in fetal alcohol syndrome and fetal alcohol effects. *Developmental and Behavioral Pediatrics* 2004; **25** (4): 228–238.

36. Steinhausen H, Spohr H. Long-term outcome of children with fetal alcohol syndrome: Psychopathology, behavior, and intelligence. *Alcoholism Clinical and Experimental Research* 1998; **22**: 334–338.

37. Famy C, Streissguth A, Unis A. Mental illness in adults with fetal alcohol syndrome or fetal alcohol effects. *American Journal of Psychiatry* 1998; **155**: 552–555.

38. Fryer S, McGee C, Matt G *et al.* Evaluations of psychopathological conditions in children with heavy prenatal alcohol exposure. *Pediatrics* 2007; **119** (3): e733–e741.

39. Blaser S, Venita J, Becker L *et al.* Neonatal brain infection. In: Rutherford M (ed). *MRI of the Neonatal Brain,* 4th edn. W.B. Saunders Ltd.: Oxford, 2001: 201–224.

40. Yamashita Y, Fujimoto C, Nakajima E *et al.* Possible association between congenital cytomegalovirus infection and autism disorder. *Journal of Autism and Developmental Disorders* 2003; **33** (4): 455–459.

41. Libbey J, Sweeten T, McMahon W. Autistic disorders and viral infections. *Journal of Neurovirology* 2005; **11**: 1–10.

42. Chess S, Korn S, Fernandez P. *Psychiatric Disorders of Children with Congenital Rubella*. Brunner/Mazel: New York, 1971.

43. Lim KO, Beal DM, Harvey RL. Brain dysmorphology in adults with congenital rubella plus schizophrenia-like symptoms. *Biological Psychiatry* 1995; **37** (11): 764–776.

44. Brown AS, Cohen P, Harkkavy-Friedman J *et al.* Prenatal rubella, premorbid abnormalities, and adult schizophrenia. *Biological Psychiatry* 2001; **49** (6): 473–486.

45. Mednick SA, Machon RA, Huttunen MO *et al.* Adult schizophrenia following prenatal exposure to an influenza epidemic. *Archives of General Psychiatry* 1988; **45** (2): 189–192.

46. Brown A, Begg M, Gravenstein S. Serologic evidence for prenatal influenza in the etiology of schizophrenia. *Archives of General Psychiatry* 2004; **61**: 774–780.

47. Moreno JL, Kurita M, Holloway T *et al.* Maternal influenza viral infection causes schizophrenia-like alterations of 5-HT1A and mGlu1 receptors in the adult offspring. *The Journal of Neuroscience: The Official Journal of the Society for Neuroscience* 2011; **31** (5): 1863–1872.

48. Brown A, Schaefer C, Quesenberry C *et al.* Maternal exposure to toxoplasmosis and risk of schizophrenia in adult offspring. *American Journal of Psychiatry* 2005; **162**: 767–773.

49. Mellins CA, Brackis-Cott E, Leu CS *et al.* Rates and types of psychiatric disorders in perinatally human immunodeficiency virus-infected youth and seroreverters. *Journal of Child Psychology and Psychiatry and Allied Disciplines* 2009; **50** (9): 1131–1138.

50. Rice F, Jones I, Thapar A. The impact of gestational stress and prenatal growth on emotional problems in the offspring: A review. *Acta Psychiatrica Scandinavica* 2007; **115**: 171–183.

51. Rice F, Harold GT, Boivin J *et al.* The links between prenatal stress and offspring development and psychopathology: Disentangling environmental and inherited influences. *Psychological Medicine* 2010; **40** (2): 335–345.

52. Hunter SK, Mendoza JH, D'Anna K *et al.* Antidepressants may mitigate the effects of prenatal maternal anxiety on infant auditory sensory gating. *American Journal of Psychiatry* 2012; **169** (6): 616–624.

53. Van den Bergh BR, Van Calster B, Smits T *et al.* Antenatal maternal anxiety is related to HPA-axis dysregulation and self-reported depressive symptoms in adolescence: A prospective study on the fetal origins of depressed mood. *Neuropsychopharmacology* 2008; **33**: 536–554.

54. Halligan SL, Murray L, Martins C *et al.* Maternal depression and psychiatric outcomes in adolescent offspring: A 13-year longitudinal study. *Journal of Affective Disorders* 2007; **97**: 145–154.

55. Karg K, Burmesiter M, Shedden K *et al.* The serotonin transporter promoter variant (5-HTTLPR), stress and depression meta-analysis revisited: Evidence of genetic modulation. *Archives of General Psychiatry* 2011; **68** (5): 444–454.

56. Khashan AS, McNamee R, Henrikson TB *et al.* Risk of affective disorders following prenatal exposure to severe life events: A Danish population-based cohort study. *Journal of Psychiatric Research* 2011; **45**: 879–885.

57. Welberg LA, Seckl JR. Prenatal stress, glucocorticoids, and the programming of the brain. *Journal of Neuroendocrinology* 2001; **13**: 113–128.

58. Seckl JR, Meaney MJ. Glucocorticoid programming. *Annals of the New York Academy of Sciences* 2004; **1032**: 63–84.

59. Rahman A, Bunn J, Lovel H *et al.* The association between antenatal depression and low birth weight in a developing country. *Acta Psychiatrica Scandinavica* 2007; **115**: 481–486.

60. Brown AS, Susser ES. Prenatal nutritional deficiency and risk of adult schizophrenia. *Schizophrenia Bulletin* 2008; **34** (6): 1054.

61. Whitaker AH, Feldman JF, Lorenz JM *et al*. Neonatal head ultrasound abnormalities in preterm infants and adolescent psychiatric disorders. *Archives of General Psychiatry* 2001; **68** (7): 742–752.

62. Whitaker AH, Van Rossem R, Feldman JF. Psychiatric outcomes in low-birth-weight children at age 6 years: Relation to neonatal cranial ultrasound abnormalities. *Archives of General Psychiatry* 1997; **54** (9): 847–856.

63. Pasamanick B, Rogers ME, Lilienfield AM. Pregnancy experience and the development of behavior disorders in children. *American Journal of Psychiatry* 1956; **112** (8): 613–618.

64. Botting N, Powls A, Cooke R *et al*. Attention deficit hyperactivity disorders and other psychiatric outcomes in very low birth weight children at 12 years. *Journal of Child Psychology and Psychiatry* 1997; **38** (8): 931–941.

65. Bhutta AT, Cleves MA, Casey PH *et al*. Cognitive and behavioral outcomes of school-aged children who were born preterm. *Journal of the American Medical Association* 2002; **288** (6): 728–737.

66. Lindström K, Lindblad F, Hjern A. Preterm birth and attention-deficit/hyperactivity disorder in schoolchildren. *Pediatrics* 2011; **127** (5): 858–865.

67. Pinto-Martin JA, Levy SE, Feldman JF *et al*. Prevalence of autism spectrum disorder in adolescents born weighing <2000 grams. *Pediatrics* 2011; **128** (5): 883–891.

68. Geddes JR, Lawrie SM. Obstetric complications and schizophrenia: A meta-analysis. *The British Journal of Psychiatry* 1995; **167** (6): 786–793.

69. Dalman C. Signs of asphyxia at birth and risk of schizophrenia: Population-based case-control study. *The British Journal of Psychiatry* 2001; **179** (5): 403–408.

70. Beauchaine TP, Hinshaw SP, Gatzke-Kopp L. Genetic and environmental influences on behavior. In: Beauchaine TP, Hinshaw SP (eds.). *Child and Adolescent Psychopathology*. John Wiley & Sons, Inc.: New Jersey, 2008: 58–92.

71. Mittal VA, Ellman LM, Cannon TD. Gene-environment interaction and covariation in schizophrenia: The role of obstetric complications. *Schizophrenia Bulletin* 2008; **34** (6): 1083–1094.

72. Rosso IM, Cannon TD. Obstetric complications and neurodevelopmental mechanisms in schizophrenia. In: Cicchetti DC, Walker EF (eds.). *Neurodevelopmental Mechanisms in Psychopathology*. Cambridge University Press: Cambridge, 2003: 111–137.

73. Duncan LE, Keller MC. A critical review of the first 10 years of candidate gene-by-environment interaction research in psychiatry. *American Journal of Psychiatry* 2011; **168** (10): 1041–1049.

74. McGowan PO, Sasaki A, D'Alessio AC *et al*. Epigenetic regulation of the glucocorticoid receptor in human brain associates with childhood abuse. *Nature Neuroscience* 2009; **12** (3): 342–348.

75. Bagot RC, Meaney M. Epigenetics and the biological basis of gene x environment interactions. *Journal of the American Academy of Child and Adolescent Psychiatry* 2010; **49** (8): 752–771.

76. Caspi A, Sugden K, Moffitt TE *et al*. Influence of life stress on depression: Moderation by a polymorphism in the 5-HTT gene. *Science* 2003; **301** (5631): 386–389.

77. Caspi A, Hariri AR, Holmes A *et al*. Genetic sensitivity to the environment: The case of the serotonin transporter gene and its implications for studying complex diseases and traits. *American Journal of Psychiatry* 2010; **167** (5): 509–527.

78. Wankerl M, Wüst S, Otte C. Current developments and controversies: Does the serotonin transporter gene-linked polymorphic region (5-HTTLPR) modulate the association between stress and depression? *Current Opinion in Psychiatry* 2010; **23** (6): 582–587.

79. Caspi A, Moffitt TE, Cannon M *et al*. Moderation of the effect of adolescent-onset cannabis use on adult psychosis by a functional polymorphism in the catechol-O-methyltransferase gene: Longitudinal evidence of a gene X environment interaction. *Biological Psychiatry* 2005; **57** (10): 1117–1127.

80. Caspi A, McClay J, Moffitt TE *et al.* Role of genotype in the cycle of violence in maltreated children. *Science* 2002; **297** (5582): 851–854.

81. Kim-Cohen J, Caspi A, Taylor A *et al.* MAOA, maltreatment, and gene-environment interaction predicting children's mental health: New evidence and a meta-analysis. *Molecular Psychiatry* 2006; **11** (10): 903–913.

82. Reif A, Rösler M, Freitag CM *et al.* Nature and nurture predispose to violent behavior: Serotonergic genes and adverse childhood environment. *Neuropsychopharmacology: Official Publication of the American College of Neuropsychopharmacology* 2007; **32** (11): 2375–2383.

83. Kloke V, Jansen F, Heiming RS *et al.* The winner and loser effect, serotonin transporter genotype, and the display of offensive aggression. *Physiology & Behavior* 2011; **103**: 565–574.

84. Taylor SE, Way BM, Welch WT *et al.* Early family environment, current adversity, the serotonin transporter polymorphism, and depressive symptomatology. *Biological Psychiatry* 2006; **60**: 671–676.

85. Belsky J, Jonassaint C, Pluess M *et al.* Vulnerability genes or plasticity genes? *Molecular Psychiatry* 2009; **14**: 746–754.

86. Harlow HF, Zimmerman RR. The development of affective responsiveness in infant monkeys. *Proceedings of the American Philosophical Society* 1958; **102**: 501–509.

87. Bowlby J. The nature of the child's tie to his mother. *International Journal of Psychoanalysis* 1958; **39**: 350–371.

88. Bowlby J. *Attachment and Loss: Volume 1: Attachment.* Basic Books: New York, 1969.

89. Ainsworth MD, Blehar MC, Waters E *et al. Patterns of Attachment: A Psychological Study of the Strange Situation.* Lawrence Erlbaum: Hillsdale, NJ, 1978.

90. Fries ABW, Ziegler TE, Kurian JR *et al.* Early experience in humans is associated with changes in neuropeptides critical for regulating social behavior. *Proceedings of the National Academy of Sciences of the United States of America* 2005; **102** (47): 17237–17240.

91. Fries ABW, Shirtcliff EA, Pollak SD. Neuroendocrine dysregulation following early social deprivation in children. *Developmental Psychobiology* 2008; **50** (6): 588–599.

92. Jones NA, Mize KD. Touch interventions positively affect development. In: L'Abate L (ed). *Low-Cost Approaches to Promote Physical and Mental Health: Theory, Research and Practice.* Springer-Verlag: New York, 2008; 353–370.

93. Johnson DE, Aronson JE, Federici R *et al.* Profound, global growth failure afflicts residents of pediatric neuropsychiatric institutes in Romania. *Pediatric Research* 1999; **45**: 126A.

94. Smyke AT, Koga SF, Johnson DE *et al.* The caregiving context in institution-reared and family-reared infants and toddlers in Romania. *Journal of Child Psychology and Psychiatry, and Allied Disciplines* 2007; **48** (2): 210–218.

95. Fox NA, Hane AA. Studying the biology of human attachment. In: Cassidy J, Shaver PR (eds.). *Handbook of Attachment: Theory, Research, and Clinical Applications*, 2nd edn. Guilford Press: New York, 2008: 217–240.

96. Feng X, Wang L, Yang S *et al.* Maternal separation produces lasting changes in cortisol and behavior in rhesus monkeys. *Proceedings of the National Academy of Sciences of the United States of America* 2011; **108** (34): 14312–14317.

97. Suomi S. Touch and the immune system in rhesus monkeys. In: Field T (ed). *Touch in Early Development.* Lawrence Erlbaum: Mahwah, NJ, 1995: 53–65.

98. Harmon K. How important is physical contact with your infant? *Scientific American.* http://www.scientificamerican.com/article.cfm?id=infant-touch (accessed 11 September 2011).

99. Albers LH, Johnson DE, Hostetter MK *et al.* Health of children adopted from the Soviet Union and Eastern Europe: Comparison with preadoptive medical records. *Journal of the American Medical Association* 1997; **278**: 922–924.

100. Goldfarb W. Variations in adolescent adjustment of institutionally reared children. *American Journal of Orthopsychiatry* 1947; **17**: 449–457.

101. Bos K, Zeanah CH, Fox NA *et al.* Psychiatric outcomes in young children with a history of institutionalization. *Harvard Review of Psychiatry* 2011; **19** (1): 15–24.

102. Winnicott DW. *The Child, the Family, and the Outside World.* Perseus Publishing: Cambridge, MA, 1987.

103. Prescott JW. Deprivation of physical affection as a primary process in the development of physical violence. In: Gil DG (ed). *Child Abuse and Violence.* AMS Press: New York, 1979: 66–137.

104. Prescott JW. Somatosensory affectional deprivation (SAD) theory of drug and alcohol use. In: Lettieri DJ, Sayers M, Pearson HW (eds.). *Theories on Drug Abuse: Selected Contemporary Perspectives.* National Institute on Drug Abuse, Department of Health and Human Services: Rockville, MD, 1980: 286–296.

105. Pederson CA. Biological aspects of social bonding and the roots of human violence. *Annals of the New York Academy of Sciences* 2004; **1036**: 106–127.

106. Erikson EH. *Childhood and Society.* W.W. Norton & Co.: New York, 1950.

107. Erikson EH. *Identity: Youth and Crisis.* W.W. Norton & Co.: New York, 1968.

108. Ainsworth MDS, Bell SM, Stayton DJ. Infant-mother attachment and social development: Socialization as a product of reciprocal responsiveness to signals. In: Richards M (ed). *The Integration of the Child into a Social World.* Cambridge University Press: London, 1974: 9–135.

109. Schaffer HR, Emerson PE. The development of social attachments in infancy. *Monographs of the Society for Research in Child Development* 1964; **29** (3): 5–75.

110. Andrea N, Kirkland J. Maternal sensitivity: A review of attachment literature definitions. *Early Child Development and Care* 1996; **120**: 55–65.

111. De Wolff M, van Ijzendoorn MH. Sensitivity and attachment: A meta-analysis on parental antecedents of infant attachments. *Child Development* 1997; **68**: 571–591.

112. Main M, Kaplan N, Cassidy J. Security in infancy, childhood, and adulthood: A move to the level of representation. *Monographs of the Society for Research in Child Development* 1985; **50** (1–2): 66–104.

113. Murray L. The impact of postnatal depression on infant development. *Journal of Child Psychology, Psychiatry and Allied Disciplines* 1992; **33**: 543–561.

114. Crockenberg SB. Infant irritability, mother responsiveness, and social support influences on the security of infant-mother attachment. *Child Development* 1981; **52** (3): 857–886.

115. Gillath O, Shaver PR, Baek JM *et al.* Genetic correlates of adult attachment style. *Personality and Social Psychology Bulletin* 2008; **34** (10): 1396–1405.

116. Ooi YP, Ang RP, Fung DSS *et al.* The impact of parent-child attachment on aggression, social stress and self-esteem. *School Psychology International* 2006; **27** (5): 552–566.

117. Fonagy P, Target M, Gergely G. Attachment and borderline personality disorder. A theory and some evidence. *Psychiatric Clinics of North America* 2000; **23** (1): 103–122, vii–viii.

118. Bowlby J. *The Making and Breaking of Affectional Bonds.* Tavistock: London, 1979.

119. Steele H, Steele M, Fonagy P. Associations among attachment classifications of mothers, fathers, and their infants. *Child Development* 1996; **67** (2): 541–555.

120. Gallo LC, Smith TW, Ruiz JM. An interpersonal analysis of adult attachment style: Circumplex descriptions, recalled developmental experiences, self-representations, and interpersonal functioning in adulthood. *Journal of Personality* 2003; **71** (2): 141–181.

121. Grossmann K, Grossmann KE. The impact of attachment to mother and father at an early age on children's psychosocial development through young adulthood. In: Tremblay RE, Barr RG, Peters RDeV *et al.* (eds.). *Encyclopedia on Early Child Development [online].* Centre of Excellence for Early Child Development: Montreal, Quebec, 2009: 1–8.

122. Priel B, Shamai D. Attachment style and perceived social support: Effects on affect regulation. *Personality and Individual Differences* 1995; **19** (2): 235–241.

123. Piaget J. *The Construction of Reality in the Child.* Basic Books: New York, 1954.

124. Akhtar S. Object constancy and adult psychopathology. *International Journal of Psychoanalysis* 1994; **75**: 441–455.

125. Mahler MS. On the significance of the normal separation-individuation phase: With reference to research in symbiotic child psychosis. In: Schur M (ed). *Drives, Affects and Behavior*, Vol. II. International Universities Press, Inc.: New York, 1965: 161–169.

126. Burland JA. Splitting as a consequence of severe abuse in childhood. *Psychiatric Clinics of North America* 1994; **17** (4): 731–734.

127. Aschersleben G, Hofer T, Jovanovic B. The link between infant attention to goal-directed action and later theory of mind abilities. *Developmental Science* 2008; **11** (6): 862–868.

128. Meins E. The effects of security of attachment and material attribution of meaning on children's linguistic acquisitional style. *Infant Behavior and Development* 1998; **21** (2): 237–252.

129. Fonagy P, Target M. Attachment and reflective function. *Development and Psychopathology* 1997; **9**: 679–700.

130. Sharp C, Fonagy P, Goodyear IM. Imagining your child's mind: Psychosocial adjustment and mothers' ability to predict their children's attributional response styles. *British Journal of Developmental Psychology* 2006; **24**: 197–214.

131. Meins E. *Security of Attachment and the Social Development of Cognition*. Psychology Press: Hove, 1997.

132. Stern DN. Mother and infant at play: The dyadic interaction involving facial, vocal and gaze behaviors. In: Lewis M, Rosenblum LA (eds.). *The Effect of the Infant on Its Caregiver*. John Wiley & Sons, Inc.: New York, 1974.

133. Stern DN. *The Interpersonal World of the Infant: A View from Psychoanalysis and Developmental Psychology*. Basic Books: New York, 1985.

134. Stern DN. Affect attunement. In: Call JD, Galenson E, Tyson RL (eds.). *Frontiers of Infant Psychiatry*, Vol. II. Basic Books: New York, 1985: 3–14.

135. Ornstein PH. Chronic rage from underground: Reflections on its structure and treatment. In: Cooper AM (ed). *Contemporary Psychoanalysis in America: Leading Analysts Present Their Work*. American Psychiatric Publishing, Inc.: Washington, DC, 2006: 449–463.

136. Kohut H. Thoughts on narcissism and narcissistic rage (1972). In: Ornstein PH (ed.). *The Search for the Self*, Vol. II. International Universities Press, Inc.: New York, 1978: 615–658.

137. Stern DN. *Diary of a Baby: What Your Child Sees, Feels, and Experiences*. Basic Books: New York, 1990.

138. Fonagy P, Gergely G, Jurist E *et al*. *Affect regulation, Mentalization, and the Development of the Self*. Other Press: New York, 2002.

139. Gergely G, Fonagy P, Target M. Attachment, mentalization, and the etiology of borderline personality disorder. *Self Psychology* 2002; **7** (1): 61–72.

140. Beebe B, Stern DN. Engagement-disengagement and early object experiences. In: Freedman M, Grand S (eds.). *Communicative Structures and Psychic Structures*. Plenum Press: New York, 1977: 35–55.

141. Beebe B, Sloate P. Assessment and treatment of difficulties in mother-infant attunement in the first three years of life: A case history. *Psychoanalytic Inquiry* 1982; **1** (4): 601–623.

142. Wallin DJ. *Attachment in Psychotherapy*. Guilford Press: New York, 2007.

143. Lyons-Ruth K. Implicit relational knowing: Its role in development and psychoanalytic treatment. *Infant Mental Health Journal* 1998; **19** (3): 282–289.

144. Stern DN, Sander LW, Nahum JP *et al*. Non-interpretive mechanisms in psychoanalytic psychotherapy: The "something more" than interpretation. *International Journal of Psychoanalysis* 1998; **79**: 903–921.

145. Beebe B, Lachman F. *Infant Research and Adult Treatment: Co-constructing Interactions*. Analytic Press: Hillsdale, NJ, 2005.

146. Lewis M, Volkmar F. *Clinical Aspects of Child and Adolescent Development*. Lea and Febiger: Philadelphia, 1990: 170–192.

147. Freud S. Three essays on the theory of sexuality. In: Strachey J (ed). *The Standard Edition of the Complete Psychological Works of Sigmund Freud, Volume VII (1901–1905): A Case of Hysteria, Three Essays on Sexuality and Other Works*, Hogarth Press: London, 1905: 123–246.

148. Sophocles. *The Three Theban Plays*. Penguin Books: New York, 1982.

149. Freud S. Letter 46 extracts from the Fliess papers. In: Strachey J (ed). *The Standard Edition of the Complete Psychological Works of Sigmund Freud, Volume I (1886–1899): Pre-Psycho-Analytic Publications and Unpublished Drafts*, Hogarth Press: London, 1896: 265.

150. Isay R. *Being Homosexual: Gay Men and their Development*. Farrar Straus Giroux: New York, 1989: 29–30.

151. Anisfeld L, Richards AD. The replacement child: Variations on a theme in history and psychoanalysis. *Psychoanalytic Study of the Child* 2000; **55**: 301–318.

152. Freud S. The neuro-psychoses of defence. In: *The Standard Edition of the Complete Psychological Works of Sigmund Freud, Volume III (1893–1899): Early Psychoanalytic Publications*. Hogarth Press: London, 1962: 41–61.

153. Moore BE, Fine BD. *Psychoanalytic Terms and Concepts*. Yale University Press: New Haven, 1990: 133–135.

154. Roiphe H, Roiphe A. *Your Child's Mind*. St. Martin's Press: New York, 1985.

155. Erikson E. *Childhood and Society*, 2nd edn. W.W. Norton & Co.: New York, 1963.

156. Piaget J. *The Child's Conception of the World*. Harcourt, Brace: New York, 1929.

157. Leventhal BL, Dawson K. Middle childhood: Normality as integration and interaction. In: Offer D, Sabshin M (eds.). *Normality and the Life Cycle: A Critical Integration*. Basic Books: New York, 1984: 30–75.

158. Rubin Z. *Children's Friendships*. Harvard University Press: Cambridge, MA, 1980.

159. Espelage DL, De La Rue L. School bullying: Its nature and ecology. *International Journal of Adolescent Medicine and Health* 2011; **24** (1) 3–10.

160. Friedman RC, Downey JI. *Sexual Orientation and Psychodynamic Psychotherapy: Sexual Science and Clinical Practice*. Columbia University Press: New York, 2002.

161. Pruitt D. *Your Adolescent*. HarperCollins: New York, 1999.

162. Walsh BT. Eating disorders. In: Tasman A, Kay J, Lieberman JA, *et al.* (eds.). *Psychiatry*, 3rd edn. Wiley-Blackwell: Chichester, 2008: 1609–1625.

163. Kosten TR. General approaches to substance and polydrug use disorders. In: Tasman A, Kay J, Lieberman JA, *et al.* (eds.). *Psychiatry*, 3rd edn. Wiley-Blackwell: Chichester, 2008: 957–970.

164. Suarez-Orozco C. Understanding and serving the children of immigrants. *Harvard Educational Review* 2001; **71** (3): 579–589.

165. Newcomb MD, Scheier LM, Bentler PM. Effects of adolescent drug use on adult mental health: A prospective study of a community sample. *Experimental and Clinical Psychopharmacology* 1993; **1**: 215–241.

166. Valliat GE. *Aging Well: Surprising Guideposts to a Happier Life from the Landmark Harvard Study of Adult Development*. Little, Brown and Company: New York, 2003.

PART FOUR: LINK

Introduction

> ### Key concepts
>
> The final step in constructing a psychodynamic formulation is to LINK the problems and patterns to history to form hypotheses about a person's development.
> To LINK, we
>
> - focus what we have DESCRIBED and REVIEWED to hone in on the patient's greatest areas of difficulty and most problematic aspects of development
> - LINK these using organizing ideas about development.
>
> When we write psychodynamic formulations, our language should indicate that the links we make are hypotheses, not facts.
> The way we LINK ultimately guides the treatment.

By this point in the book, you've learned how to describe problems and patterns and how to take a thorough developmental history. But, as we've said in Chapter 1, when we formulate, we do more than report histories – we form hypotheses about how a person's history might have led to the development of his/her unique problems and patterns. To think about this, let's recall the example of Ms A from Chapter 2, the 43-year-old woman who came for treatment with Dr Z because she was worried that her husband would leave her. As Dr Z conducted the evaluation, she learned that despite Ms A's considerable talents, Ms A was unable to say anything good about herself. This incongruity caused Dr Z to wonder why Ms A had this view of herself. Then, when Dr Z took the developmental history, she learned that Ms A's mother was a world-famous scientist who was critical of her daughter's complete lack of interest in science, preferring Ms A's brother who became a physicist. Dr Z then formed an early formulation (hypothesis) that Ms A had unconscious, maladaptive ways of perceiving herself and regulating her self-esteem that might have developed as the result of her problematic relationship with her mother.

How did Dr Z form this hypothesis? It was not magic. Rather, as she learned about Ms A's problems and patterns, she asked herself a question:

Why does this talented woman have such a low opinion of herself?

Because she was thinking psychodynamically, she DESCRIBED Ms A as having difficulties with self-esteem regulation that likely reflected unconscious, overly critical perceptions about herself and her abilities. This gave Dr Z a partial answer to her question, but she knew that in order to develop a strategy for helping Ms A with her low self-esteem, she would need to understand how and why these unconscious, maladaptive self-perceptions had developed. To answer that, Dr Z REVIEWED Ms A's developmental history and, among other things, learned that she had had a difficult relationship with her critical, dismissive mother. She then used an organizing idea about development – that maladaptive self-perceptions are often related to a person's early relationship with a dismissing, critical parent – to LINK the pattern to the history. By describing, reviewing, and linking, she had formed an hypothesis about why Ms A had such a low opinion of herself – a psychodynamic formulation.

Focusing the formulation

This example, written to clearly illustrate this process, is overly simplified. It's easy for Dr Z to LINK patterns and history because, as far as we see, Ms A presents only one pattern and only one aspect of her history. In real clinical situations, however, the process is much more complex. As you've read throughout this book, people think, feel, and do myriad things, and their histories are long and complicated. There's no possible way that we can form hypotheses about every aspect of their functioning or link every moment in their histories to the way they developed. But even more importantly, this would not necessarily be helpful. The primary goal of the formulation is to guide the treatment. A diffuse, overly inclusive formulation will not help to give us direction in the treatment, but a **focused formulation** will. Preparing to link involves focusing what we have DESCRIBED and REVIEWED to hone in on the most important "dots to connect." Here's how we can do this:

focus DESCRIBE

Once we have a sense of the person's overall function, we need to focus on the aspects that we think are most important to understand. These are generally the areas that are giving the person the greatest difficulty. A helpful tool is trying to ask a **focus question**, which we can think of as the question that we would most like to answer with our psychodynamic formulation. Let's think about this using two brief examples:

> *Mr B is a 50-year-old man who presents saying that he is having trouble at work. He says that although he does excellent work, his boss is "out to fire" him. He says that this "always happens at jobs – the people seem OK at first, but then you realize that they're just like everybody else – it's each man for himself." Mr B has no friends and lives alone. "Investing in other people is for chumps," he tells the therapist.*

> *Mr C is a 50-year-old man who presents saying that he is having trouble at work. He enjoys his job, but is unsure that it's what he really wants to do in life. "I've been doing this for years, and I'm good at it, but is it my life passion? I'm so confused." He says that, during early adulthood, he went into the same career as his brothers without thinking, but he now wonders, "Maybe I should do something else for the second half of my life. But what?"*

Mr B and Mr C both present with trouble at work; however, Mr B's greatest difficulty seems to be his inability to **trust** others (focus question: "Why can't Mr B trust other people?"), while Mr C's greatest difficulty seems to be in the area of **identity** (focus question: "Why is Mr C so unsure about what he wants to do in life?") Despite the surface similarity of their complaints, their areas of greatest difficulty are very different. Our questions, our formulations, and our treatments will thus be very different for Mr B and Mr C.

Although it may not always be possible, it's worth trying to focus on one, or at most two, areas. This may be harder when people have global difficulties; then, a focus question may be "Why does this person have difficulty in so many aspects of his/her life?"

focus REVIEW

As with DESCRIBE, once we have a sense of the person's overall history, it's time to focus – this time, on the points in development that were most likely to have disrupted or supported healthy development. Traumas, separations, problematic relationships, and emotional/cognitive difficulties are likely to disrupt development, while secure relationships, the absence of trauma, and good cognitive function are likely to support healthy development. Summarizing the highlights – both problematic and growth supporting – of each phase of life gives us a bird's-eye view of the developmental history and provides valuable clues for linking the history to the problems and patterns.

When considering how to focus on key moments in development, remember that global problems with function tend to arise earlier, while more circumscribed problems tend to arise later (see the Introduction to Part Three). This is not *always* true because protective factors such as resilience and later developmental repair (like new relationships and psychotherapy) can mitigate the affect of early problems, but it is still useful to consider.

LINK using organizing ideas about development

Finally, we need to connect the major difficulties to the key points in the person's developmental history. This is the all-important step – the point at which we turn the history into a formulation – the moment when we commit to an idea about causation. For this crucial step, we rely on **organizing ideas about development**. These organizing ideas are ways of conceptualizing how what happens during development could lead to the problems and patterns that we see in our adult patients. They help us to answer questions like

> *How might early trauma lead to problems with affect regulation?*
>
> *How might depression in childhood lead to problems with self-esteem management?*
>
> *How might an absent mother lead to interpersonal problems in adulthood?*
>
> *How might having an attuned mother help someone to grapple with a breakup in college?*
>
> *How might an overly close relationship with a parent lead to sexual inhibitions?*

There are many different ideas about development that can help us to link a person's developmental history to his/her adult patterns of thinking, feeling, and behaving. Each idea offers a different way to explain how a person's history – including nature and nurture – could result in the problems and patterns that we see in the adult. We can link problems and patterns to history by thinking about the impact of

- trauma
- early cognitive and emotional difficulties
- conflict and defense
- relationships with others
- the development of the self
- early attachment patterns.

When we LINK, we scroll through these organizing ideas to choose the ones that will help us to make useful connections between the patient's patterns and the developmental history. We can use several ideas for a single formulation, and we can use different ideas in different formulations. Each chapter in Part Four presents one of these organizing ideas about development so that you can begin to have a library of ideas to choose from when you construct your formulations.

So many organizing ideas – how do we choose?

Just as there are many ideas about development, there are many ways to link a patient's patterns to his/her history. The way the clinician does this in a psycho-dynamic formulation depends on many variables, including the way the patient tells his/her story and the needs of the clinical situation. There are some clinical situations that are well explained using particular organizing ideas about development, and we outline such situations with examples in each of the chapters in this part. Nevertheless, it generally makes sense to lead with the information from the description and the history and *then* to choose ideas about development, rather than beginning with a favorite idea. Try to avoid "looking for history" that suits an idea about development – this can skew the formulation. For example, consider two people with difficulty regulating affect, one who had an abusive parent and one who had early bipolar disorder – despite the similarly of their difficulties, their psychodynamic formulations might require two different ideas about development.

Writing a psychodynamic formulation

Even though not all psychodynamic formulations are written, we suggest trying to write some chronological narratives as you learn to DESCRIBE, REVIEW, and LINK. As you write, think about how things that happened early in life might have affected later development – for example, how problems with self-esteem from the earliest years might have affected identity consolidation in adolescence, how the trust consolidated during a primary dyadic relationship might have helped someone through a later trauma, or how problems with competition from middle childhood might have affected career development in young adulthood. Start with a summary that outlines your focal points, then try to comment on the way the person developed during each phase of life. At the end of Part Four, you can listen in as one therapist considers how to "put together" a full psychodynamic formulation, and you can then read his narrative.

When you write *your* formulations, remember that the links we make between history and adult patterns are hypotheses – best guesses based on developmental research and empirical work with patients. They are not facts. They are designed to help us to understand our patients, to help our patients understand themselves, and to guide our treatments. Thus, the language of linking should reflect this. When we link, we use words like "perhaps" and "maybe" and phrases like "it could be" and "it is likely that." Saying

> *Mr D's problems with self-esteem were caused both by his chronic mood disorder and by his lack of acknowledgment by his father.*

is very different than saying

> *Mr D's report of both a lifelong history of low mood and a consistent lack of mirroring by his father suggests that these may have contributed to the development of his difficulties maintaining and managing self-esteem.*

The second way makes it clear that the links between Mr D's difficulties with self-esteem and the elements of his history are hypotheses, not established facts.

Using ideas about development over time

As you gain comfort with formulating, you will not necessarily always consciously think about and apply different ideas about development. They will become a part of the way you automatically think about patients. However, while you are learning to formulate, we suggest that you carefully consider all of these organizing ideas with each patient to decide which ones can best help you to form hypotheses about the individual's development.

Linking guides treatment

The way we link our adult patients' problems and patterns to their unique histories guides our treatment. If we link adult problems to early trauma, we need to help our patients understand their traumatic experiences and repair disrupted development. If we link problems to unconscious conflicts and defenses, we need to help our patients develop more adaptive ways of dealing with them. If we link problems to relationships with others, we need to help our patients develop new relationship templates. Our formulations guide our goals for treatment, the way we listen to our patients, and the way we choose our interventions (see Chapter 3). Generally, we can help our patients by (1) making them aware of a problematic aspect of their development or function and (2) helping them to develop new, healthier function. We discuss this in each of the chapters in this part of the book.

Looking ahead

In each of the chapters in Part Four, we present one organizing idea about development, outlining

- the basics of the organizing idea
- clinical situations for which the organizing idea is particularly useful
- a sample formulation using the idea
- ways in which linking to that idea guides treatment.

Note that our sample formulations in these chapters present DESCRIBE and REVIEW sections that have already been focused and thus only contain the major difficulties and key developmental points.

Now, let's move on to our first organizing idea about development – linking problems and patterns to trauma.

Suggested activity

Consider Mr A and Ms B. What would you focus on as the major difficulty or difficulties of each, and why? What might be a focus question?

Mr A is a 29-year-old man who is living with his girlfriend. He presents for therapy saying that he's not sure whether he should break up with her. He says that she is trying to control his life with endless demands on his time and that she doesn't understand what men need. He also complains that in the last few months, she has only wanted to have sex twice a week. Mr A is an unsuccessful solo entrepreneur. "I can't stand working with other people," he explains, "Most people are idiots." When the therapist suggests that perhaps his girlfriend just enjoys spending time with him, he says, "I can't believe you would say that. Haven't you been listening?"

Comment

Mr A seems to have difficulty with **mentalization** and **empathy**. He is unable to imagine that either his girlfriend or his therapist could have thoughts and feelings that are different from his. It also impairs his ability to have a good sense of self and others. Possible focus questions include "Why can't Mr A think about the thoughts and feelings of others?" and "Why does Mr A lack empathy?"

Ms B is a 21-year-old college student. She presents with anxiety around doing assignments for her college courses. She has close relationships with her parents, and she has many good friends, several of whom try to help her with her work. "I just can't keep it all straight," she says, "I end up with paper all over the room, and I never know what to start with." She did well in high school, albeit with several tutors. She cannot relax, and her stress is taxing her friendships.

Comment

Ms B likely has difficulty with **cognition**. Although testing might be required to understand the exact nature of the difficulty, it could be a learning disability, or a problem with decision making or organizing her work. Her trouble with relaxation and friendships seems to be clearly connected to her primary cognitive problem. A possible focus question might be "Why does Ms B have so much difficulty keeping herself organized?"

13 Trauma

Key concepts

When trauma is prominent in a person's history, we may be able to LINK the development of the adult's problems and patterns to the impact of trauma.

Trauma is an experience of extraordinarily stressful and disturbing events that overwhelms the individual.

Trauma can affect the development of all aspects of functioning.

Linking to the impact of trauma is particularly useful when constructing case formulations for patients who have problems with

- self-experience
- affect regulation and impulse control
- adapting to stress
- forming and maintaining secure attachments

Human experience has always been colored by traumatic events, ranging from personal traumas, such as childhood abuse and neglect, to cataclysms affecting whole populations, such as the Holocaust, the events of September 11, and natural disasters. We take for granted that traumatic experiences have a psychological effect on people. But why is this true? Ideas about the impact of trauma on development can help us make the link between traumatic events in a person's history and his/her characteristic problems and patterns.

What is trauma?

Psychological trauma can be defined as the experience of extraordinarily stressful, disturbing, or violent events, over which the victim is helpless and which overwhelm his/her psychological and biological capacity to cope [1, 2]. DSM-IV defines traumatic events as those in which "the person experienced, witnessed, or was confronted with an event or events that involved actual or threatened death or serious injury, or a threat to the physical integrity of self or others," and the response to these events involves intense fear, helplessness, or horror [3]. Trauma can involve a single event or experience, or a protracted period of suffering or victimization.

Psychodynamic Formulation, First Edition. Deborah L. Cabaniss, Sabrina Cherry, Carolyn J. Douglas, Ruth L. Graver, and Anna R. Schwartz.

Basic ideas about how trauma can affect development

People who study mental health have long grappled with the question of how trauma affects development. One of the earliest psychodynamic ideas about this was Freud's hypothesis that childhood sexual abuse could lead to physical or "conversion" symptoms in adulthood [4]. Just as there is no single type of trauma, there is no single idea about how trauma shapes a person's characteristic problems and patterns. In addition, all current theories suggest that there is no one-to-one correlation between trauma and psychological difficulties. Multiple variables may affect how people process traumatic events:

- **Extent and severity of trauma** – Extreme and protracted traumatic experiences, such as internment in a concentration camp, severe physical and sexual abuse in childhood, or prolonged combat exposure, are likely to leave lasting psychic scars on the victims. More circumscribed traumatic events, such as surviving a natural disaster, a severe accident, or a violent crime, may have more variable outcomes.

- **Age at which trauma occurs** – Trauma in childhood affects the developing brain and can cause global disruption of function. It is associated not only with post-traumatic stress disorder (PTSD) and other anxiety disorders but also with mood disorders, affective dysregulation, attachment disorders, substance abuse, and problems with academic performance and social relationships [5–10]. Childhood abuse has been correlated with abnormalities in neural systems involved in regulation of affect and response to stress [11–16]. Animal studies suggest that early maternal loss or deprivation of care can disrupt neural systems that are normally regulated by close physical and emotional contact between infant and mother, resulting in lasting perturbations in stress response systems and increased susceptibility to stress and disease later in life [17, 18].

- **Resilience** – It is not known why trauma affects some individuals more or in different ways than it does others. For example, the prevalence of PTSD is lower than that of trauma itself [19, 20]. Individual differences in vulnerability and resilience in the face of trauma may reflect neural and/or genetic predispositions and may influence the likelihood of developing symptoms of PTSD [21, 22].

PTSD, as it is currently defined by the DSM-IV, captures only some aspects of human response to trauma, namely, a specific set of symptoms involving reexperiencing the traumatic event(s), avoidance and numbing, and hyperarousal. Researchers in this area have proposed that a new diagnostic category be created, called **complex PTSD**, which more fully describes the impact of protracted trauma on self-experience, self-regulation, and relationships with others [2, 23]. This disorder, also referred to as Disorders of Extreme Stress Not Otherwise Specified (DESNOS), posits that people with a childhood history of repeated interpersonal trauma manifest a typical pattern of problems with regulation of affect and impulses, memory and attention, self-perception, interpersonal relations, somatization, and systems of meaning [24]. The debate over the validity of DESNOS as a diagnostic category is beyond the scope of this book, yet when we are constructing psychodynamic formulations it is useful to remember how pervasive the impact of trauma can be.

Linking problems and patterns to the impact of trauma

Whenever there is a history of trauma, using ideas about the way trauma affects development can help us to link history to adult problems and patterns. When we formulate using ideas about the impact of trauma on development, we trace problems and patterns to the individual's reactions to traumatic events and situations. Here are some clinical situations for which linking to trauma is particularly useful:

Problems with self-experience

Particularly when trauma occurs early in life and involves chronic abuse at the hands of parents or trusted adults, traumatized children may experience significant impairment in the development of a coherent and stable sense of self. Children who have been the victims of abuse tend to blame themselves, rather than accept the fact that their caregivers are unreliable, exploitative, or violent. Such misattribution of blame may reflect the cognitive limitations of a young child and may also be a way of trying to make sense of an otherwise terrifying situation. This may persist and lead to self-deprecating or masochistic patterns in the adult (see Chapter 4). The deep feelings of guilt and shame that often accompany trauma can persist into adulthood and profoundly affect self-esteem [23, 25].

Trauma that occurs in adulthood can disrupt a previously well-established sense of self [26, 27]. Even when it occurs later in life, trauma may result in a sense of having two distinct experiences of oneself and the world: the "traumatic" and the "nontraumatic," or the "before-the-trauma" and the "after-the-trauma" perspectives – these may be difficult to integrate.

Example

Mr A is a 32-year-old man who sought psychotherapy for long-standing problems with self-esteem and difficulty forming romantic relationships. He describes chronic feelings of being an "outsider," different from the rest of his family and most peer groups. He feels easily ashamed, humiliated, or guilty, particularly when he experiences himself as not living up to his own very high standards or when he is unsuccessful socially. He and his therapist have been exploring possible origins of these patterns in his early family life. Mr A was a quiet, bright, and motivated student, unlike his parents and siblings, who were extroverted and athletic and did not emphasize intellectual pursuits. Although his family members are quite religiously observant, Mr A stopped attending church during college and considers himself an atheist. Six months into psychotherapy, Mr A discloses to his therapist that, from the ages of 9 to 11, a clergyman in his family's church sexually abused him. He says that he has been too ashamed to discuss this with anyone, but realizes that many of the painful feelings he has been exploring originated during this time.

The problems and patterns with which Mr A struggles may have multiple roots in development. However, the experience of having been sexually abused by a trusted adult, along with years of harboring a shameful secret, is likely to have intensified his feeling of "otherness" and his difficulty with self-esteem.

Problems with regulation of affect and impulses

Trauma can also lead to persisting problems with regulation of affect and impulse control. As described, traumatic stress during childhood is associated with the development of psychiatric symptoms and disorders in adulthood, including depression, suicidality, PTSD and other anxiety disorders, and personality disorders, as well as difficulties regulating anger and sexual impulses [7–9, 28].

Patients with PTSD often suffer either from intense emotional and physical hyperarousal or from emotional blunting or numbing. In patients who do not necessarily meet the PTSD criteria, or who have a trauma history that is unacknowledged, these forms of affective dysregulation may be diagnosed as a primary affective disorder or borderline personality disorder. Judith Herman, in her landmark book, *Trauma and Recovery*, argues that many patients diagnosed with borderline personality disorder have histories of abuse and that the affective lability seen in that disorder may be better conceptualized as the aftereffects of chronic trauma [2].

Another clinical phenomenon seen in trauma survivors that may be linked to trauma-induced affective dysregulation is deliberate self-harm or self-mutilation. Typically involving cutting or burning of the skin, this behavior is more common in those with a childhood abuse history and often serves the purpose of relieving states of emotional distress, such as anxiety, depression, or dissociation [28, 29].

Example

Ms B is a 23-year-old woman who is referred for ongoing psychiatric treatment after a brief hospitalization following a suicide attempt. She describes overwhelming feelings of hopelessness and despair following a breakup with her boyfriend that led her to impulsively swallow a bottle of her roommate's antidepressant medication. Ms B reports that since early adolescence, she has had a history of "mood swings," alcohol and drug abuse, skin cutting, and bulimia. Despite these symptoms, Ms B has worked as a computer programmer since graduating from college a year ago. She describes a history of repeated sexual abuse by her stepfather between the ages of 6 and 12. He warned her that if she ever told anyone about "their secret" he would kill her. Years later, after her mother and stepfather had separated, Ms B finally told her mother what had happened. While she was being abused, Ms B had frequent physical complaints and performed poorly in school. She started experimenting with drugs in early adolescence and had multiple sexual partners. Ms B describes her emotional life as "a roller coaster," alternating between extremes of anger, sadness, or anxiety and numbness or emptiness. Unaccustomed to talking about her feelings or personal thoughts, she says she usually "takes action" to handle painful emotions.

The experience of protracted sexual abuse early in life may have affected Ms B's ability to tolerate and regulate painful or uncomfortable feelings. Being forced to keep her experiences secret may have led her to adapt to stress by acting rather than talking. This trauma-informed approach to psychodynamic formulation is very useful in clinical situations such as in Ms B's.

Problems with interpersonal relationships

Traumatic experiences can also affect the ability to establish relationships with others in a variety of ways. The ability to trust is particularly vulnerable to trauma that is perpetrated by others. Early childhood abuse, especially if at the hands of a family member or caregiver, can affect the developing child's ability to form secure attachments (see Chapter 18) [5, 6, 10]. In normal development, children's interactions with caregivers who are consistent, loving, and empathic lay the groundwork for healthy relationships in later life. Children whose caregivers were violent or neglectful, or who were unable to protect them from other violent adults (e.g., during wartime), may be unable to trust others and form secure attachments. As adults, they may have difficulties along a continuum from a pervasive sense of mistrust or paranoia to more circumscribed problems with intimacy (see Chapter 5).

Example

Mr C, an 85-year-old man, is referred to the clinic when he refuses to have further diagnostic studies to evaluate a suspicious nodule on his chest X-ray. Mr C tells the psychiatrist that he knows it could be cancer, but says, "If it's cancer, what could they do for me? There's no help for that, so why should I find out?" Mr C's son, who has accompanied him to the appointment, says that his father will never ask for help or rely on others and that he prides himself on his business successes as a self-made man. As a young child during World War II (WWII), Mr C remembers their neighbors watching as the Nazis dragged the family out of their apartment and sent them to a concentration camp. In the camp, he was separated from his parents and siblings, all of whom were killed.

Mr C, who survived the Holocaust and built a successful life for himself as an adult, has a deep-seated belief that other people cannot help him or save him from danger. The horrible reality of his early life makes it difficult for him to believe that people in the present may be able to help him. Linking Mr C's difficulty with trust to his early trauma is a useful way to construct a formulation about his development.

Problems with adapting

Difficulty adapting to stress can often be usefully linked to trauma. In fact, one of the hallmarks of PTSD is an abnormal set of responses to external stimuli. Patients with PTSD may be hyperreactive to stimuli that remind them of traumatic experiences, for example, the sound of a low-flying airplane or a car backfiring. What might be "ordinary" stress for a nontraumatized individual is often experienced as extraordinary stress for someone with a trauma history. For example, a child who grew up repeatedly witnessing her mother being beaten by her father might be especially averse to any kind of interpersonal conflict. A child who had to flee her home and country due to war may respond with great distress to separation from important people and places as an adult.

Example

Ms D, a recently divorced mother of a 2-year-old daughter, presents for treatment complaining of severe insomnia, anxiety, and difficulty functioning at work. She describes "falling apart" after her husband of 5 years left her for another woman soon after their child was born. Ms D feels she should be "coping better" with the divorce and says, "I'm not as strong as my mom was after she left my dad." Ms D's father physically abused her mother and her older brother for several years until her mother fled not only from her husband but also the country, emigrating illegally to the

United States with her two children when Ms D was 7 years old. Ms D says that although she knew that her father was violent, she also has memories of feeling very attached to him as a young child. She says she's always had difficulty with separation from people she's close to.

Ms D's current experience of loss and betrayal in her marriage echoes the earlier traumas of domestic violence, family disruption, and emigration. Understanding this link is helpful in understanding her current difficulties.

Childhood abuse can also disrupt the development of object constancy (see Chapter 10), leading to a reliance on splitting-based defenses later in life. By splitting off the negative aspects of an abusive or a neglectful caregiver, mistreated children can continue to believe in the goodness of those on whom they depend, albeit at a high cost. This tendency may persist into adulthood and lead to maladaptive responses to stress and interpersonal conflict [28, 30, 31].

Example

For the first three months of their relationship, Mr E thought that his girlfriend was "the best thing that ever happened to him." However, after she canceled a date because she had to babysit for her divorced sister's children, Mr E decided that she was a "horrible liar" and immediately broke up with her. As a child, Mr E lived with his father after his mother abandoned them. Although his father was alcoholic and extremely neglectful, he idealizes him as "the man who saved my life" and joined with his father's vitriolic attacks on his mother.

Abandoned by his mother and dependent on his neglectful father, Mr E needed to deny his father's mistreatment in order to feel that someone cared for him. This has likely led to his persistent use of splitting-based defenses that do not allow him to have nuanced views of others. Rigid and sustained use of maladaptive defenses can often be usefully understood as stemming from trauma.

A sample formulation – linking to trauma

Presentation

Ms F is a 44-year-old woman who seeks psychotherapy for long-standing difficulties maintaining relationships with other people and chronic feelings of low self-esteem. She says that she would like to have a long-term relationship with a man, and perhaps marry, but although her romantic relationships always start out passionately, they have never lasted longer than a year. Although she has an active social life, with many acquaintances, Ms F says, "I don't have any real friends, there's no one I can confide in." She describes herself as "naïve" when it comes to choosing friends and lovers, saying, "I keep picking the wrong people who turn out to be really manipulative, cruel, and selfish." She tends to end relationships abruptly once she feels betrayed or rejected. Ms F has "tried therapy" several times in the past, but became disillusioned or angry with each therapist after a few months. At the end of the second session she tells the therapist, "I can tell you're different than the other therapists I've seen – you're really smart and you understand me perfectly."

DESCRIBE the problems and patterns (*focused*)

*Ms F has difficulty maintaining **relationships with others**. She has trouble with **intimacy**, rapidly entering into intense but shallow relationships with friends and lovers, and then becoming quickly and easily hurt or angry. She has a poor **sense of self and others** and at times is unable to tolerate the slightest imperfection or shortcoming in other people. She often chooses people who take advantage of her desperate-seeming need to connect, and thus, her relationships lack **mutuality**. She is overly **trusting** of people who give her little reason to have confidence in them. The short-term quality of her relationships suggests that her attachments are generally **insecure**.*

REVIEW the developmental history

Ms F is the only child of a mother who was diagnosed with schizophrenia when Ms F was in her mid-teens, and who has been intermittently psychotic for most of Ms F's life. Her father worked long hours and was often absent from home. Ms F describes her mother as being "different people at different times." While she was sometimes loving and attentive, she could also be violent and abusive, shouting insults or obscenities at Ms F, locking her in her room for long periods of time and often hitting her. The family lived in near isolation, with no extended family and infrequent contact with friends or neighbors.

LINK the history and problems/patterns to the impact of trauma

Ms F's difficulty maintaining relationships with others may be related to her trouble integrating good and bad qualities in herself and others. This may have resulted from her traumatic childhood experiences with her mother. Her mother's wildly inconsistent and frightening behavior made it hard for Ms F to develop a well-functioning internal sense of herself in relation to a generally consistent and positive other. Ms F may have needed to keep good and bad aspects of her mother separate in her mind to adapt to the bewildering fluctuations in her mother's behavior. Her tendency to gravitate to people who are cruel or emotionally abusive may be related to expectations, instilled in her by childhood experiences, that abuse is the price one has to pay for having some sense of safety and security with others.

Linking to trauma guides treatment

Understanding the relationship between a patient's problems/patterns and history of trauma is crucial for formulating a diagnosis and treatment plan. Patients can benefit enormously from being able to discuss their experiences with a mental health professional who can listen to them in an empathic, nonjudgmental way. Often, we are the first people with whom our patients discuss their traumatic experiences. If we give them time, their stories will generally emerge bit by bit. By acknowledging the effects that trauma may have had on them, and showing that we can bear to hear about it, we can establish an atmosphere of safety and trust that is crucial in helping them begin therapy. Over time, their trust in us may also help them to increase their general ability to trust, form secure attachments, and have a more integrated sense of self and others. Sharing our formulations with them may increase their understanding of the way their traumatic experiences have affected their current functioning.

Example

Ms G is a 28-year-old administrative assistant who presents for an evaluation after developing anxiety attacks. She just started a new job and tells the therapist that she feels intimidated by her boss, a man in his 60s. She feels jumpy and on edge at work, has lost her appetite, and often wakes up in the middle of the night after nightmares. Ms G's father was verbally and occasionally physically abusive to his children, and Ms G and her siblings walked on eggshells around him, never knowing what might set off his temper. The therapist asks Ms G whether the way she feels in the presence of her new boss is similar to how she felt around her father, and she says, "Yes, I have that same scared feeling that he might yell at me at any moment."

Linking Ms G's experience of traumatic fear in childhood to her current situation may give her a way of understanding her current emotional responses and help her to find new ways of adapting.

Suggested activity

How would you describe the ways in which the two people described below have reacted to the traumas they experienced?

Ms A is a 75-year-old Jewish woman who comes to see you for mild depression. She retired from her job six years ago, feels a bit lost and unsure of her role in life, and would like to talk about how to feel better. She has four children and 12 grandchildren and is involved in all of their lives. Ms A was born in an Eastern European country. When she was 7 years old, her family was arrested by the Nazis and sent to a concentration camp. Her parents and older brother died in the camp, but she and her sister survived. The camp was liberated by Allied forces, and Ms A and her sister emigrated to the United States when she was 12 years old. When Ms A retired from her job, she decided that she wanted to write a memoir about her experience in the Holocaust. Her survival was a miracle, she says, and life is a gift. She felt it was important to record the events she witnessed and that writing about them would help her to integrate her early experience with who she is now. She enrolled in several writing courses, which she enjoyed and where she met interesting people. She asks if you would like to read her memoir sometime.

Mr B is a 75-year-old man who is brought to you by his wife for consultation. She says that her husband has been depressed all his life, but in the past year it has gotten much worse. She says he barely speaks to her, rarely leaves the house, and spends most of his time reading books about history. Mr B says, "Of course I'm depressed, look at the life I've had. What's the point of talking about it? I just want everyone to leave me alone." Mr B was born in an Eastern European country, to Jewish parents. When he was 6 years old, the family tried to flee the country to escape the Nazi invasion, but they were captured and sent to a concentration camp. His parents were killed, but he and a younger brother survived. They immigrated to the United States several years later. Mr B says that although he married, had children, and became a successful businessman, he feels that he spent his whole life pretending to be a "normal person." He says that he believes life has no meaning, he can't trust anyone except his wife, and there is no hope for his future.

Comment

Although both Ms A and Mr B have similar histories of almost unimaginable trauma, their reactions to their experiences have been very different. Each has developed depression in later life, though Ms A's depression is much less severe than Mr B's. Each is struggling with questions about purpose and meaning in life but approaches them with very different attitudes. These differences may arise from their response to early traumatic experiences, which may in turn stem from their innate temperaments, capacities for resilience, and early relationships with others. Ms A seems to have the ability to trust (including the possibility of trusting that a therapist can help her), form attachments, maintain positive self-esteem, enjoy work and play, and have a sense of hope. Mr B, on the other hand, does not trust others, has a severely impaired capacity for pleasure, is unable to be hopeful, and lacks a coherent sense of self. If possible, it would be helpful to learn about their early lives and relationships prior to the trauma, although the effects of trauma on memory often make this difficult.

14 Early Cognitive and Emotional Difficulties

Key concepts

Understanding the way our patients' early cognitive and emotional difficulties affected the development of their conscious and unconscious thoughts, feelings, and behavior can help us to LINK problems and patterns to their history.

Cognitive and emotional difficulties are very common in childhood and adolescence and can disturb whatever development is occurring at that time. They include problems that both do and do not meet the criteria for DSM disorders.

The response of caregivers and early treatment can alter the extent to which cognitive and emotional difficulties affect development.

Adult patients may not be aware that early cognitive and emotional difficulties played a role in their development, particularly when they were not recognized or treated. We should consider linking problems and patterns to early cognitive and emotional difficulties when

- there is an apparent "mismatch" between what we describe and what we review
- there is a history in childhood or adolescence of a sudden delay or unexpected interruption in previously normal development
- there is a personal or family history of cognitive and emotional difficulties

As we discussed in Chapter 9, when we construct psychodynamic formulations we generally think about the way in which people's interactions with others, particularly early caregivers, shaped their adult problems and patterns. However, like adults, children and adolescents have problems with mood and anxiety, as well as other cognitive and emotional difficulties, that can profoundly affect their development. Some of these may be diagnosed and treated, but many are not; in fact, adults who had these kinds of problems may never have conceptualized them in this way. Nevertheless, as we construct our psychodynamic formulations, we have to remain alert to the possibility that a problem of this nature may have been a factor in our patients' early lives. In this chapter, we review some of the cognitive and emotional difficulties that commonly occur during childhood and adolescence and then suggest clinical situations for which linking to them may be helpful.

Psychodynamic Formulation, First Edition. Deborah L. Cabaniss, Sabrina Cherry, Carolyn J. Douglas, Ruth L. Graver, and Anna R. Schwartz.
© 2013 John Wiley & Sons, Ltd. Published 2013 by John Wiley & Sons, Ltd.

Why talk about difficulties rather than disorders?

While some of the cognitive and emotional difficulties that people have during development reach the level of being a disorder, many do not. Think of the child who tends to procrastinate during elementary school but who does not meet the criteria for attention deficit disorder (ADD), or the teenager who is often sad but does not meet the criteria for major depression or dysthymia. Despite the fact that they are not disorders, these difficulties can have a major impact on the development of all aspects of function, including self-experience, relationships with others, adapting, cognition, and work/play. Consequently, we think that it is important to broadly consider the impact of our patients' cognitive and emotional **difficulties** as well as their frank disorders.

Basics related to the impact of cognitive and emotional difficulties on development

Cognitive and emotional difficulties are quite common in children and adolescents. Data on a representative population of American children growing up in the 1990s showed that about one in three had at least one psychiatric disorder by age 16 [32], and, frequently, they had more than one psychiatric diagnosis [33–35]. Among all adults with psychiatric illness, about three-quarters had received a diagnosis before age 18 and half before age 14 [36–38].

Whenever cognitive and emotional difficulties occur, they have the capacity to disturb development happening during that period, as well as functioning that will develop later. For example, difficulties in later childhood that interfere with performing school tasks and developing friendships with peers (such as ADD or childhood bipolar disorder) are powerful predictors of poor work ethic in adulthood [39, 40]. Thus, when we hear that someone has a history of cognitive and emotional difficulties in childhood or adolescence, it's important to determine exactly when those problems emerged, what should have been developing during those periods, and whether those problems may have compromised aspects of later development.

To think about this further, let's consider some specific cognitive and emotional difficulties that arise during different phases of development:

Cognitive and emotional difficulties in childhood

Cognitive and emotional difficulties that commonly emerge during the childhood years (0–12) include [32, 36]

- autism spectrum disorders
- academic/learning difficulties (including learning disorders)
- attentional difficulties (including ADHD)
- anxiety (including OCD, phobias, and separation anxiety disorder)

- enuresis/encopresis
- motor/verbal tics
- mood difficulties (including depression)

Some of these difficulties may even begin at birth and be related to inherited disorders, prenatal development, or temperamental traits (see Chapter 9). When they begin in early childhood (before age 6), they can have profound and pervasive effects on emotional, cognitive, and physical development and may predict a lifetime of problems, especially in the absence of early detection and intervention [41]. For example, early, undiagnosed depression, as well as subthreshold mood disorders, can affect everything from the development of self-esteem to relationships with others. Recognizing that these problems may have been at play can help us to understand our patients and can help our patients to better understand themselves.

Example

Ms A is a 32-year-old single computer-aided design draftsman who is referred by her employee assistance program because of recent conflicts with coworkers. With a somewhat flat affect, she says that she enjoys her job preparing topographical maps for civil engineering projects but has trouble relating to peers and supervisors. She has no friends, has never been in a romantic relationship, and her only activity outside of work is folding complicated origami designs. Ms A reports that, since earliest childhood, she has always been "the odd man out": "My mother said I was a late talker and was just reserved – she said the other kids would understand me better when I got older. It never happened."

We can hypothesize that Ms A's social awkwardness, developmental delays, and odd interests might be related to a previously unrecognized autism spectrum disorder such as Asperger's syndrome. This link can help us to understand her difficulty getting along with others and having mutually satisfying adult relationships.

The ways in which children adapt to their cognitive and emotional difficulties can further affect development. For example, learning disabilities or ADHD may compromise school performance, self-esteem, and the ability to form friendships. If children then isolate themselves to avoid social rejection, they may compound the effect of the original problem:

Example

Mr B is a 46-year-old single school bus driver who was referred by his supervisor after screaming at children on the bus. Until recently, he enjoyed his job driving younger kids to school but he began to have trouble when asked to take on a new route for high-school students. Despite having grown up in a supportive, middle-class family, Mr B reports that he had a "miserable" childhood plagued by learning disabilities, expressive language problems, and ADHD. Mr B states that he never developed "conversational techniques" and had virtually no friends. In high school, as other classmates began dating, Mr B tended to avoid social interactions and his provocative remarks and "holier-than-thou" attitude further alienated peers.

Mr B's inability to adapt to his learning disabilities during childhood may have compromised the development of his sense of self and contributed to his patterns of responding to self-esteem threats with avoidance and grandiosity.

Cognitive and emotional difficulties in adolescence

Across cultures and centuries, adolescence has always been a time of dramatic change in body and behavior. During the teen years, enormous changes also take place in the neural systems that control higher cognitive functions, interpersonal interactions, self-regulation, and motivation. As such, it is a time of high risk since brain systems appear to be most vulnerable when they are evolving – as one author suggested, "moving parts get broken" [42, 43].

Despite bumps in the road, most adolescents eventually manage to navigate the transition from dependent children to self-sufficient young adults. However, the turbulent teen years can be even more challenging if the adolescent is also contending with cognitive and emotional difficulties. Problems that typically emerge or worsen during adolescence include difficulties with [32, 36, 37]

- anxiety (including panic disorder, generalized anxiety disorder, and PTSD)
- eating (including anorexia nervosa and bulimia)
- conduct (including conduct and oppositional defiant disorders)
- emotional regulation and impulse control
- mood (including major depression and bipolar disorder)
- psychosis (including schizophrenia)
- substance abuse

Adolescents with difficulties in any of these areas may miss out on the opportunity to develop and strengthen the skills their peers are practicing, including the ability to regulate affect, control impulses, exercise self-restraint, and consolidate identity (see Chapter 12). They may continue to have trouble in these areas even during periods when their cognitive and emotional difficulties are less problematic.

Example

Ms C is a 53-year-old woman who presents for help with "figuring out what I want to do with my life." She says for the past 18 years she has been a stay-at-home mom, but that since her youngest daughter went to college last year, she has been bored at home and is thinking about doing something else. However, she is unclear about her interests and has no particular skills. This is making her feel "like a failure." When the therapist reviews Ms C's developmental history, she learns that although Ms C was a very good student in elementary school, she spent most of high school and college battling anorexia. She recovered after an inpatient stay in her early 20s and has been normal weight ever since. She explains, "Then I got married and started having kids, and now I'm here."

When other adolescents and young adults were consolidating their identities and building careers, Ms C was dealing with anorexia. Although she has been free from symptoms for over 25 years, she is left without a clear sense of what she enjoys doing and without skills that might help her negotiate the next phase of her life.

Cognitive and emotional difficulties in adulthood

Although our focus in this chapter is on the impact of cognitive and emotional difficulties in childhood and adolescence, development doesn't stop at age 18 (see Chapter 12). Thus, emotional and cognitive difficulties that arise in adulthood can also affect development.

Example

Ms D is a 35-year-old married mother of a 4-year-old son, who presents because she is afraid of having a second child. Although she reports that she and her husband want more children, she says, "I don't think that I'm a good at this. I don't think that I can handle taking care of babies. And it's so lonely." When the therapist asks more about her experience of having had her son, Ms D explains that she spent "weeks home crying alone" after her son was born. "It was miserable. I just felt so incompetent. I've always been confident and good at what I've done – but I'm not good at this."

In this situation, it is likely that Ms D had an untreated postpartum depression. This has left her feeling that she is a terrible mother and fearful about having a second child. These are new patterns that evolved in adulthood, which we can usefully link to the effects of a problem with mood on her sense of self.

Parental response and early treatment can help mitigate the impact of cognitive and emotional difficulties on development

The extent to which early cognitive and emotional difficulties impact development depends on various factors, including [44–47]

- the nature, timing, and chronicity of the difficulty
- the child's early relationship with primary caregivers, including the caregivers' responsiveness to the difficulty
- general family stress and the child's social environment
- peer relationships
- parental socioeconomic status, which can affect access to resources
- adequate early treatment, and the way the difficulty is conceptualized by the caregivers and, ultimately, by the child.

Parental response to a child's cognitive and emotional difficulties and early treatment intervention can make an enormous difference in the way those problems impact development [48].

Example

Ms E, a 30-year-old happily married teacher, presents for "grief counseling" following the sudden death of her mother. She denies any previous history of mental health treatment. She tells her therapist that she understands why she is feeling such wrenching grief, but says that she is troubled by the near-panic-like anxiety that has gripped her since the funeral: "It's like my first day at nursery school and Mom is walking out the door." Asked what she recalls about that day, Ms E says that she has a vivid memory of entering the classroom and throwing herself on the ground and screaming, even after the teacher reassured her that her mother could stay for a while. Her mother consulted a child psychologist who worked with her to develop a plan to return Ms E to school as quickly as possible. Within a few weeks, Ms E waved happily and turned back to play with the other children when her mother told her she was "just taking a quick coffee break." "It's hard to believe I couldn't let my mother out of my sight back then," Ms E remarks, "When it came time to apply to college, my first choice was St. Andrew's in Scotland."

In Ms E's case, early and aggressive behavioral treatment, sensitive parenting, and a supportive school environment all contributed to limiting the duration and impact of her early separation anxiety. It is important to remember that although positive responses from caregivers and early recognition/treatment may help mitigate negative consequences, they are not necessarily protective against the disruptive effects of these early difficulties, particularly when they reach the level of being psychiatric disorders.

Linking problems and patterns to the impact of early cognitive and emotional difficulties

Although some patients can tell us that they had early cognitive and emotional difficulties, many cannot. How, then, can we know when to usefully hypothesize about links to early emotional problems? Some guidelines that can help us with these questions are presented in the following.

"Mismatch" between what we describe and what we review

Sometimes, what we describe and what we review just don't seem to match. For example, someone may present with global disruption of function but describe having grown up in a very supportive, functional early environment with siblings who do not have the same difficulties. Or patients might describe having had "terrible" caregivers who "ruined" their lives but again this might not seem to match what you learn about the caregivers over time. Although it is always possible that one member of the family is treated differently from the others, it is also possible that the patient may have had an early cognitive or emotional problem. Of course, it's not always one or the other – a child with early difficulties may, in fact, be treated differently from other children in the family, either with more or less attention, empathy, and patience.

Example

Ms F is a 21-year-old college student who is referred by her college dean after roommates noticed that she had multiple cuts on her arm. Ms F admits that she started cutting herself "again" after discovering that her boyfriend was communicating with other women via social networking. She says, "I've always been all over the place – up, down – I don't know what's wrong with me. Nothing bad ever happened to me – my parents are good people who try to help but they just don't get where I came from – my brother and sister never had these problems. Why can't I get it together?"

Ms F's pervasive problems with mood and self-mutilation, in the setting of what sounds like a "good enough" family situation, suggests that she has likely been suffering from lifelong problems with mood and self-regulation. Understanding this can help her not only to get appropriate treatment but also to have a new understanding of her development that can help her improve her self-esteem and relationships with others.

History in childhood of unexpected interruption of previously normal development

Hearing about sudden or unexpected interruptions in a previously normal develop-ment should trigger the thought that early cognitive or emotional difficulties may have played a role. Consider Mr G:

Mr G is a 35-year-old man who presents for help negotiating social issues in his new company. "I started at a small firm, and this is a real step up – but the place is huge! I feel a little lost and don't know how to find good mentors." Although Mr G denies current symptoms of anxiety or depression, he admits to feeling a little "off-kilter." When the therapist reviews the developmental history, Mr G describes having been an excellent student, with many friends, "Except for sixth and seventh grade. I don't know what happened – I was in a new school and I just imploded or something. I spent all of my time in my room playing video games. My grades plummeted. My parents were constantly angry with me – telling me to 'get on the stick.' But by eighth grade I was OK again. Maybe it was the new school. That experience has always made me worried about new situations."

The sudden interruption of function in later childhood, with social isolation and disruption of school performance, suggests that Mr G might have had a mood disorder – perhaps an undiagnosed major depression – at the beginning of middle school. However, this is not the way he or the people around him conceptualized it. The episode led to conflicts with his parents and affected his confidence about entering new situations. Linking Mr G's current problem to this early emotional difficulty can enhance our understanding of the way Mr G developed his patterns of self-esteem regulation and relationships with others.

Personal or family history of cognitive and/or emotional difficulties

It almost goes without saying that early cognitive and emotional difficulties should be suspected as contributing to the current problems and patterns when there is a personal or family history of this, as in the following example:

Ms H is a 28-year-old physical therapist and a mother of two who presents saying that she needs help trying to feel better about herself. "Everyone at work is smarter or more interesting than I am," she says, "And I need to be stronger when my husband gives me a hard time." Ms H denies current symptoms of depression, but says that she was always a "quiet" child who kept to herself. She did not volunteer for things at school, and she generally presumed that she would not be chosen for school plays and sports teams. "I'm kind of like my mom," she says, "She was pretty low energy." Although she doesn't know the details, she says that she thinks that her maternal grandmother once took something for depression.

Although Ms H does not complain of depression, her family history suggests that some difficulties with mood – either depression or dysthymia – may have played a role in her development. This has likely affected the way she consolidated her sense of self and her ability to manage self-esteem.

A sample formulation – linking to the impact of early cognitive and emotional difficulties

Linking problems and patterns to the impact of early cognitive and emotional difficulties is about more than making diagnoses – it's about trying to understand the ways that those early problems impacted our patients' development, including their conscious and unconscious ways of thinking about themselves, relating to others, adapting to stress, thinking, working, and playing. When you suspect that an early cognitive or emotional problem existed, don't stop there – think about the way it affected both the person and the person's environment throughout development. Here's an example:

Presentation

Ms I is a 45-year-old married part-time legal secretary who comes in with her husband saying that she is "exhausted." She explains that she "had to quit" her job because it's "too much." Her husband explains that Ms I has quit a series of temp jobs that she'd taken on since he went on disability for a back injury a year ago. Previously, Ms I had been supported by her husband and never worked outside the home. Her husband complains she is "acting like a sad sack" and is "lazy and unmotivated" – "She knows what she needs to do and if she'd quit surfing the net at work, she'd be great, but she won't do the work unless she wants to." Interviewed alone, Ms I states that she had been "keeping up OK" at work at first, but when she was asked to cover several partners and things became more hectic, she felt increasingly depressed and anxious, was unable to concentrate, slept poorly at night, felt tired and apathetic on awakening, and had trouble getting to work on time. She feels ashamed and frustrated about her "collapse" but can't understand why she keeps "losing it" – "I'm just one of those people who can't seem to get it together."

DESCRIBE (*focused*)

Problem

Ms I is overwhelmed by tasks at work, leading her to quit jobs repeatedly. She has particular difficulty staying focused and organized, and she finds it hard to prioritize tasks, tending to flit from one thing to the next without finishing anything. In the wake of having quit her most recent job, she is also feeling depressed and anxious, with some difficulty sleeping. Ms I is also having difficulty in her relationship with her husband, who thinks that she quitting her jobs because she is lazy.

Patterns

Ms I identifies herself as a "housewife" and states that she has no trouble keeping up with household tasks, shopping, and paying bills "as long as I take my time." She has a good sense of herself in this role but feels that she is "limited" in her abilities and intelligence. She tends to defer to her husband and often feels bullied by him. While adjusting to working outside the home has been a challenge, Ms I states she wants to "do my part" with her husband on disability and is hurt that he thinks she's unwilling to work hard. She has good female friends with whom she talks on the phone and occasionally has lunch. She has few other leisure activities – she explains, "it generally takes me twice the time to do whatever other people are able to do – so it's hard to find time to relax."

REVIEW the developmental history

Ms I is the only child born to a single mother whom she describes as "loving but depressed – she had a hard life but she did the best she could to give me a better life." Her mother worked two jobs and was rarely home for dinner but tried to make up for lost time by devoting herself to her daughter on the weekends. Ms I states that she had "always loved school" until 4th grade when she suffered a head injury in a fall while ice-skating with her mother. She doesn't recall much about the incident but was told by her mother that doctors said her X-ray reports were fine. Soon after, Ms I began to throw tantrums as her mother tried to dress her for school and was disciplined for hitting other girls. She had more trouble paying attention in class, had trouble keeping up with math, and could only read a few sentences at a time before losing track of the overall "gist" of the text. She needed help organizing herself to do home work and tended to procrastinate to the last minute before completing assignments. By the end of middle school, her exasperated mother gave up trying to motivate her and simply wrote her essays for her. Ms I started to slip into worsening depression and anxiety toward the end of high school but would not accept any psychological help. She "limped" through secretarial school, but after meeting her future husband, she was relieved that she wouldn't have to look for a job.

LINK the history and problems/patterns to the impact of early cognitive and emotional difficulties

Ms I's current work-related difficulties are likely related to long-standing cognitive problems, which may date back to an episode of head trauma in childhood that was never defined or treated. Ms I's cognitive difficulties have likely contributed to her lifelong difficulties with self-esteem, including her feelings of intellectual inferiority, and have likely impaired her relationships with others. Her contentious relationship with her mother may have stemmed from her cognitive problems but may also have contributed to the development of poor self-perceptions and difficulty with self-esteem management. All of these are likely to have contributed to her choice of spouse, as well as her choice to remain at home.

Linking to early cognitive and emotional difficulties guides treatment

If we suspect that a person's development and current difficulties may have been influenced by early cognitive and/or emotional difficulties, this can influence treatment in several ways:

- further testing (e.g., neuropsychological testing) may be needed to define the nature and severity of cognitive problems
- taking a family history for cognitive and emotional difficulties should be a part of every evaluation but may need to be reviewed in greater depth if there is any suspicion that they may have affected development and contributed to the patient's current problems
- appropriate interventions for concurrent cognitive or psychiatric problems (cognitive remediation, pharmacotherapy, etc.) may be a mainstay of treatment

Recognition and acknowledgment of the presence and impact of early cognitive and emotional difficulties can offer patients the opportunity to create new and often more forgiving life narratives that can help them understand themselves in a new way. In addition, treatment of underlying difficulties, such as anxiety and depression, can often substantially improve the patient's quality of life, function, and feelings about themselves – and, with time, can help patients to develop new conscious and unconscious ways of thinking about themselves and others.

Thinking back to Ms I, let's consider how the formulation might guide the treatment:

> The therapist refers Ms I to a neuropsychologist for further testing and to a psychiatrist for evaluation of her mood and anxiety symptoms. He also offers Ms I and her husband psychoeducation, suggesting that her work-related difficulties have nothing to do with laziness or lack of effort. He explains that bright, motivated people with cognitive problems may abandon tasks not because they are lazy but because they have lost track of what they are doing, especially if they are working in a hectic, stressful environment like a busy law firm. The therapist also expresses optimism that after neuropsychological testing has helped define the nature of her cognitive problems, Ms I should benefit greatly from both cognitive remediation to improve her neuropsychological skills and psychotherapy to help her to understand the way she thinks about herself, her abilities, and her relationships with others.

In the case of Ms I, helping her and her husband understand that her work-related difficulties are related at least in part to early cognitive and emotional difficulties, rather than character flaws, may go a long way toward repairing her sense of self and lessening tensions and misunderstandings in the marriage.

Suggested activity

How might the following be linked?

1. *Ms A's difficulty asking her boss for a raise – her early temperamental shyness.*
2. *Mr B's difficulty dealing with his 8-year-old daughter – his early learning difficulties.*
3. *Ms C's difficulty with self-esteem regulation – her early encopresis.*

Comment

1. There are many reasons why Ms A might have difficulty asserting herself at work, but if she gives a history that suggests that she has been shy since her earliest years, this could definitely be a contributing factor. It could be the persistent shyness itself and/or it could also be other patterns (such as avoidance or self-deprecation) that evolved as a result of the shyness. Identifying this as a temperamental trait could be very important to the formulation and the treatment.

2. Having had a learning difficulty himself, Mr B could become irritable, anxious, or fearful as his daughter begins to do classroom work that gave (or continues to give) him difficulty. Understanding this link could help him to understand his feelings and could lead to improvement in the relationship.

3. Any early difficulty that potentially leads to shame, such as enuresis or encopresis, can affect the developing child's sense of self and capacity for self-esteem regulation. This can affect the adult's ability to regulate self-esteem long after the childhood difficulty disappears.

15 Conflict and Defense

Key concepts

An organizing idea about development, called **ego psychology**, suggests that adult problems and patterns can be LINKED to unconscious conflicts and defenses.

According to this idea, unconscious conflict happens when opposing thoughts, feelings, or wishes collide. This conflict, which is out of awareness, causes anxiety, prompting us to use defenses to work out compromises. These compromises result in our characteristic problems and patterns.

Linking the development of problems and patterns to unconscious conflicts and defenses is particularly useful for understanding difficulties related to

- competitive anxiety and inhibitions
- difficulties with commitment and sexual intimacy
- more adaptive defenses

Picture this: you're a sophomore in college, it's Saturday at 5 pm, and all of your friends are going to a party. You'd love to go, but you know that you have tons of work to do before Monday. What do you do? Part of you feels you need a break after a long week, but another part feels obligated to start that stack of homework. You waffle back and forth and finally decide to stay home. Once your friends have left the dorm, you sit down at your desk to begin. Before you start, though, you decide to clean your desk. Then your desk looks so clean in comparison to the mess around it, you decide to clean the whole room. While you're doing that, you find a note that your friend from high school called, so you call your friend back, talk for while, make yourself a sandwich, and by the time you sit down again it's 11:30 pm and you haven't done any work! What happened?

Conflict and compromise

What happened to you on that Saturday night is that you were conflicted. Part of you wanted to go out to have fun, and part of you felt that you should stay home to do your work. These two parts were in **conflict** [49, 50]. Although you thought that you

---

Psychodynamic Formulation, First Edition. Deborah L. Cabaniss, Sabrina Cherry, Carolyn J. Douglas, Ruth L. Graver, and Anna R. Schwartz.
© 2013 John Wiley & Sons, Ltd. Published 2013 by John Wiley & Sons, Ltd.

had a made a choice, the battle continued without your knowing it and your mind forged a **compromise** [50]. The compromise was that you stayed home (partially satisfying the part of your mind that felt obligated to do homework), but you didn't do any work (partially satisfying the part that wanted to relax after a long week). All of this happened out of awareness, so we call it **unconscious conflict** [49–51]. One way of thinking about the way the mind works and develops, called **ego psychology**, suggests that conflicts like this one occur constantly and underlie the way we think, feel, and behave.

Basics of ego psychology

Conflict→ Anxiety→ Defense

The idea that problems and patterns can be linked to unconscious conflict was originally conceptualized by Freud [52]. Freud first thought that the conflict was between *two* parts of the mind – the conscious part and the unconscious part. He called this idea the **topographic model** because it describes the mind as having one part (the conscious part) that is "on top of" the other part (the unconscious part) [53]. According to this idea, problems arise when unconscious thoughts and feelings are prevented from reaching consciousness, generally because they are deemed too painful to be tolerated. Freud soon realized, however, that conflict could exist between two parts of the mind that are *both* unconscious. This led him to a second idea, which he called the **structural model**, that described the mind in terms of structures rather than locations [53]. These structures are not anatomical; rather, we can think of them as clusters of functions. They are the id, the ego, and the superego:

- The **id** represents wishes and feelings that are unconscious because they tend to make people uncomfortable (e.g., anxious or ashamed). Consequently, they are repressed – that is, they are kept out of awareness.

- The **superego** represents the conscience and the ego ideal (the way people like to see themselves).

- The **ego** represents the executive function of the mind – the mediator among the id, superego, and reality. Ego functions include reality testing, defense mechanisms, and the capacity to conceptualize self and other [50].

According to this theory, these parts of the mind are in constant conflict with one another and with reality. Wishes, in the form of unconscious fantasy, are in conflict with the superego or with reality. Most of this conflict is unconscious – that is, out of awareness – but it nevertheless affects the individual's conscious life. In this model, unconscious conflict between or among these structures causes **anxiety**, which the ego tries to protect the person from experiencing. We can call this protection **defense** [50].

Defenses are the unconscious and automatic ways the mind adapts to stress (see Chapter 6). They are the coping mechanisms and internal compromises that limit a person's awareness of painful affects like anxiety, depression, and envy, and that resolve emotional conflicts [50].

More adaptive and less adaptive compromises and defenses

As in our example of the college sophomore, defenses try to partially satisfy each side of a conflict. The resulting thought, feeling, or behavior is thus a compromise. Some compromises are more adaptive than others, as in the following examples:

Example – more adaptive defense

Mr A, a 19-year-old man who is angry with his controlling father, takes up martial arts and becomes a black belt in karate. He is very proud of this accomplishment.

Mr A's unconscious conflict might look something like this:

I'm so anger with my father I could kill him	vs.	It would be wrong to hurt my own father

This conflict causes anxiety, which the ego protects against using a defense – in this case, **sublimation**. Sublimation is a very adaptive defense that allows someone to gratify an uncomfortable wish or feeling by doing something useful or socially acceptable [50]. By becoming interested in martial arts, Mr A partially gratifies his wish to attack his father by fighting with other men in a controlled way, while abiding by his superego's prohibition against actual violence toward his father. Mr A feels good about what he is doing, and thus this defense is adaptive for him.

Example – less adaptive defense

Ms B is a 42-year-old woman whose mother was very abusive. As a small child, Ms B was beaten for any angry outburst. As an adult, she maintains an idealized view of her mother but blames herself for everything and allows herself to be badly treated by others.

Ms B's unconscious conflict might look like this:

I love my mother and need to feel that she is taking care of me	vs.	I am angry because my mother is not taking care of me

Again, this conflict causes anxiety, which triggers the ego into action. Here, though, the ego uses a less adaptive defense called **splitting** that preserves good feelings about one person by completely devaluing another. Ms B needed her abusive mother, so she denied her mother's bad qualities and idealized her. However, since her mother continued to be abusive, Ms B assumed that it was her own fault. The defense allowed Ms B to love her mother while expressing her anger at herself. This is a compromise that "worked" (was adaptive) in childhood because it allowed Ms B to avoid thinking about the abuse and to lead as normal a life as possible. However, what worked in childhood becomes increasingly maladaptive in adulthood in the sense that Ms B's tendency to squelch her rage, blame herself, and attach to abusive people leaves her disconnected from her own feelings, unable to have a balanced view of herself and others, and less likely to find a more loving relationship (see Chapter 6 for more on defenses).

Linking problems and patterns to conflict and defense

When might we choose to link problems and patterns to conflict and defense? Thinking about the mind in terms of conflict and defense generally presumes that people **have** capacities that they defensively inhibit. Thus, we generally use this organizing idea about development for people who have fairly circumscribed problems that were developed after the earliest years. These people tend to be able to trust, to have a good sense of self and other, and to form secure relationships, but often inhibit themselves in terms of competitiveness and sexuality. Let's look at these clinical situations in more depth:

Competitive anxiety and inhibitions

In the three-person relationships of middle childhood, children struggle with fantasies of besting their parents and fears about consequently losing their love. This is an unconscious conflict. If it is not resolved in childhood, it may persist into adulthood, causing adults to continue to experience anxiety when they are competitive or assertive. This leads to defensive inhibitions. People can inhibit themselves in many ways – they can inhibit their relationships, their work, and their capacity to enjoy themselves. Consider the case of Ms C:

> Ms C is a 38-year-old heterosexual woman who presents for psychotherapy because she is having difficulty sustaining a relationship. The therapist notes that Ms C is wearing clothing that would be more appropriate for an older woman. Ms C also says that her father left her mother over 20 years ago for a younger woman and that her mother has been alone and depressed for many years. Ms C feels that she is her mother's best friend.

In this example, it is possible that Ms C has the following conflict:

I want a good relationship with a man	vs.	I can't have something my mother didn't have

The wish to have a relationship causes conflict, which triggers defenses that lead her to inhibit her femininity and potentially sabotage her chances of having a satisfying relationship. We can also say that she has an **overly harsh superego** that does not allow her to have something that she wants in order to punish her for unconscious wishes. This way of thinking about development links Ms C's problems with relationships to an unconscious conflict and her use of less adaptive defenses.

Difficulties with commitment and sexual intimacy

The three-person relationships of middle childhood also produce conflicts that can lead to adult difficulties with intimacy. As we discussed in Chapter 11, during normal development children have intense fantasies about their caregivers – they generally long for closeness with a desired caregiver while fearing punishment for this wish from a rival caregiver. If they receive enough gratification from the desired caregiver while also sensing that he/she has good boundaries, and if the rival caregiver allows for closeness and identification, children "resolve" these early fantasies by relinquishing these wishes and waiting for adult relationships of their own. However, if this does not happen, the early fantasies may persist into adulthood, leading to conflicts that can impede intimacy.

Example

Ms D is a 28-year-old woman who presents with marital problems, saying that her new husband, E, is upset because she does not seem interested in sex. Ms D says that she loves her husband, to whom she has been married for 1 year, and that their sex life was "great" prior to the wedding. However, she now feels "tired" every night and has frequent headaches prior to bedtime. Ms D says that she is also worried because her husband isn't making enough money and she fears that she won't be able to have the lifestyle that her father afforded her mother. Speaking of her father, Ms D says, "He's the best. Not only is he successful at work, but thank goodness he comes over to fix things in the house – E can't do any of that."

Here, we can hypothesize that Ms D's difficulties with sexual intimacy may arise from unresolved unconscious conflicts. She loves her husband, but worries that he will not be able to live up to her ideals, modeled on her own father. She may not have relinquished her early fantasies about her father, leading her to continue to compare her husband to her father. We can think about this conflict in this way:

I want to be an adult woman and have my own adult sexual relationship	vs.	I want to remain a child and have a relationship with my father

This conflict may trigger **repression** of her sexual feelings for her husband, as well as **somatization**, that further results in her avoidance of sex. Conflicts like Ms D's can also often lead men and women to have trouble committing to relationships.

Patterns related to more adaptive defenses

Patterns related to more adaptive defenses can also be usefully understood by linking them to conflicts and defenses. While more adaptive than splitting-based defenses, these defenses can nevertheless be rigid and can cause people to have problems with the way they handle emotions. For some, fear of strong affects can lead to relatively emotionless relationships, while for others it can lead to a dramatic use of emotion to avoid more frightening feelings.

Example

Ms E is a 42-year-old woman who is married, has two children, and works at a job that carries a good deal of responsibility. Her husband, while loving, has not worked in many years. Ms E begins to have various physical ailments, requiring her to go to many doctors' visits and to stay home from work. Although medical tests do not result in any findings, she persists in her feeling that she is becoming more ill. Her husband is very understanding and accompanies her to all medical visits.

We can think of Ms E as having the following conflict:

I love my husband and don't want to feel that there is anything wrong with our marriage	vs.	I resent my husband because I have to go to work every day while he just stays home and does what he wants

In this example, Ms E defends against negative feelings about her husband using **somatization**. The compromise that the defense creates allows her to continue to have good feelings about her husband while focusing attention on her and allowing her to take a break from work.

A sample formulation – linking to conflict and defense

Formulating with ego psychology means hypothesizing that problems and patterns are linked to unconscious conflicts and defenses. Here's an example:

Presentation

Mr F is a 28-year-old man who presents for treatment saying that recently he has been delaying doing important projects for work. Although he is generally able to get his work done on time, when it comes to the big presentations he "freezes up." He is acutely aware of this because he is coming up for a major review that could impact his potential for promotion. He is frustrated with this behavior and would like to change it but does not know how.

DESCRIBE the problem and patterns (*focused*)

*Mr F reports that he has had a long-standing problem with procrastination, particularly when the stakes are high. He generally is very competent and **organized** – he loves biking and routinely takes his bicycle for tune-ups, pays his taxes by the deadline, and arranges complicated vacations. He has a good job that is **well matched to his level of education**, which he **enjoys**. He has a **secure** relationship with his wife and has several **intimate** friendships. He generally uses **adaptive defenses** that tend to keep **emotions conscious and repress thoughts**, and, as above, he uses **avoidance** as a major adaptive strategy during periods of stress.*

REVIEW the developmental history

Mr F recalls having a close and warm early relationship with his mother. He says that his father loved him as well; however, he felt that his father's esteem was much more contingent on performance. "He praised me when I did well, but was really critical and sort of withdrew from me when I didn't do spectacularly." He felt that his father devalued his mother for not being "as smart as we are," and he somewhat guiltily reports that he was favored by his father over his younger sister, who excelled in sports but not academics. Mr F says that he recalls having a happy childhood and that he had many friends. He was an avid reader and enjoyed math in elementary school. He was eager to please teachers and did not use drugs or alcohol. However, once the pressure of high school and college acceptance felt real to him, he began to have difficulty completing schoolwork. Despite excellent scores on standardized testing, his grades dropped and he matriculated at a community college before transferring to a state university. He remains close to both parents – his father often wants to have lunch to discuss Mr F's future career.

LINK the history and problems/patterns to conflict and defense

Mr F's problems with procrastination seem circumscribed. He is able to plan ahead and has considerable intellectual talents. Thus, he has abilities that he seems to be inhibiting – perhaps because of unconscious conflicts and defenses. We can hypothesize that Mr F, who felt well loved by his parents, had a secure dyadic relationship and was able to learn to trust. However, he felt that his father's esteem was in danger if he did not excel. Thus, he may have developed an unconscious conflict that was something like this:

I want to excel and do well to receive praise from my father	vs.	I want to avoid situations in which I could fail, because this could mean loss of my father's love and esteem

When Mr F is in situations in which he fears that he could fail – like his senior year in high school and now in his job – this conflict produces anxiety. The anxiety leads to a maladaptive defense – avoidance. While he consciously thinks that he wants to move forward, he unconsciously prevents himself from actually doing the work because he fears that he might fail. Although this allows him to avoid the anxiety that these situations create, it also puts him in danger of sabotaging himself despite his considerable talents.

Linking to unconscious conflict and defense guides treatment

If we suggest to our patients that their problems and patterns are linked to unconscious conflicts and defenses, we need to help them to find more adaptive ways of reconciling these conflicts and defending against anxiety. We can do this in two basic ways. If they have the ability to tolerate strong affects and are relatively self-reflective, we can help them to become consciously aware of conflicts and defenses that are giving them difficulty. We call this **uncovering** [50]. On the other hand, if they cannot tolerate strong affects and are unable to self-reflect, we can help them to shift adaptive strategies without becoming aware of their unconscious conflicts and defenses. We call this **supporting**. We briefly discuss both uncovering and supporting strategies here; please refer to *Psychodynamic Psychotherapy: A Clinical Manual* [50] for a more in-depth discussion of these techniques.

Uncovering

Just because a conflict is unconscious does not mean that it disappears. On the contrary, it continues to exert its effect on the way a person thinks, feels, and behaves. However, if it is out of awareness, the person cannot use his/her logical, conscious, adult mind to forge the compromise. Instead, a compromise is formed out of awareness, based on thoughts and fears that may have originated in childhood. One of Freud's original ideas about treatment was that it was important to "make the unconscious conscious" in order to allow the conscious mind to grapple with the conflict and to create more adaptive solutions. In therapy, we do this by having patients say whatever comes to mind (**free association**) in order to allow unconscious thoughts and feelings to become conscious. Once an unconscious fantasy comes to light, it can presumably be seen as a holdover from childhood and may cease to look so frightening. A good analogy is the thing in a dark bedroom that looks like an intruder and is revealed to be a hat on a chair when the light is turned on – making things conscious helps us to see them in a more realistic way.

Example

As a child, Mr G had a minor operation that required an overnight stay in the hospital. His parents did not stay with him, and he was terrified. Thirty years later, Mr G's doctor told him that he needed a minor surgical procedure. He was ready to sign a consent form until he found out that the procedure required a one-night hospital stay. Unaware of the connection to his childhood experience, he told the surgeon that he would not sign the consent form because he thought that the procedure was unnecessary. The surgeon recommended discussing this with a therapist. When the therapist asked him about whether he'd ever been in a hospital before, he discussed his childhood experience for the first time, realized the connection, and was able to go through with the procedure.

Psychoanalysts after Freud, including his daughter Anna Freud, became aware that it often took more than just making conflicts conscious to help a person to make more adaptive compromises. They began to focus on making the compromise and defense more adaptive, rather than simply focusing on bringing the wish or fantasy into consciousness. This is called **interpreting** or **analyzing the defense**, and this type of technique is called **defense analysis**.

Example

Ms H, a 28-year-old woman who longs for a stable relationship with a man, repeatedly gets involved with men who are only interested in short-term sexual encounters. In therapy, she learns that this is a compromise between her wish for a relationship and her sexual attraction to rough and somewhat dangerous men. Her understanding of this allows her to shift her compromise and she ultimately engages in a relationship with a loving man who is interested in skydiving and motorcycle racing – continuing to gratify both sides of the conflict but in a more adaptive manner.

Supporting

When we use techniques to support, we are supporting someone who, for one reason or another, is unable to use more adaptive defenses. This could be the result of a chronic problem, such as the persisting effects of early childhood abuse or a severe mental illness, or an acute problem, such as a recent loss or a sudden medical problem. In these situations, we do not try to make the unconscious conflicts and defenses conscious; rather, we try to support the use of more adaptive defenses while decreasing the use of less adaptive defenses.

Example

Mr I, a 45-year-old man who has just lost his job, comes to treatment for problems with "anger management" after almost starting a fight with his boss on his last day of work. "I didn't want to see a shrink," he explains, "but my wife made me come. The only thing that's wrong with me is that those idiots don't know a good worker when they see one." In the course of the interview, Mr I says that he's "too good for that job," but needs it because "times are tough." "I could have gone to college," says Mr I, "but my wife got pregnant and I had to join the union. Dad was the only one in that shop who was worth anything." The therapist empathizes with Mr I and universalizes his feeling of anger at being fired, saying, "Most people get very upset when they're laid off!" She then suggests that they think together about strategies for managing his anger, particularly during these first few days of unemployment.

The therapist recognizes that Mr I is using less adaptive defenses to deal with his anger. She even imagines that powerful unconscious conflicts – relating, for example, to his conflicting wishes to surpass the success of his working-class father and to take care of his young family – might underlie the extent of the rage that he is experiencing. However, his acute loss, as well as his current lack of self-reflection, guides her to use supporting techniques such as **empathizing**, **universalizing**, and **collaborative problem solving** to help him to use more adaptive defenses.

Suggested activity

What unconscious conflicts might be affecting Mr A?

Mr A is a 32-year-old single, heterosexual lawyer who has been dating B, a 31-year-old teacher, for 5 years. Although he feels that he is "in love" and that he wants to spend his life with B, he does not feel ready to get married. B, who comes from a large family, would like to have several children and feels ready to begin. Mr A feels troubled by his inability to commit and presents for therapy to try to understand this issue. He reports that he is from a wealthy family and enjoys spending time at his family's summer home where he frequently goes sailing with his brothers. The brothers also enjoy their yearly camping trips and weekly poker games, at which they are often joined by their father. Mr A has recently been offered a promotion at work, which would offer him the ability to support a family independently, but he is concerned that this might "trap" him in a lifestyle and leave him little ability to make a career change in a few years.

Comment

Mr A says that he wants to spend his life with B but does not feel ready for marriage. In addition, he's not sure why he's having difficulty making this commitment. This suggests that one or more unconscious conflicts could be causing him to feel "stuck." His closeness to his brothers and family suggests that this could be involved. Here is one conflict that could be operating:

I want to be a grown up man and start a family of my own	vs.	I want to remain as a child with my parents and brothers

This conflict is suggested by Mr A's continued attachment to his brothers and parents. Perhaps the closeness in this family makes it difficult for Mr A to assume a role as father in a family of his own because the gratifications of being "one of the brothers" is so enormous. Here is another conflict that could be affecting Mr A:

I want to spend my life with another person	vs.	I want to remain independent

This way of thinking about Mr A's conflict emphasizes his conflicting wishes about personal autonomy and is suggested by his recent decision at work. Both could be operating simultaneously, making it difficult for Mr A to move forward in his life.

16 Relationships with Others

Key concepts

Another organizing idea about development, called **object relations theory**, LINKS problems and patterns to the unconscious repetition of early relationships with others.

According to this idea, young children take in their experiences with important caregivers through a process called **internalization**. These internalized relationship patterns, called **templates**, remain in the unconscious mind through development, affecting the way people think about themselves and others.

Linking to unconscious relationship templates is particularly useful for understanding problems that adults have in forming relationships, including

- global problems involving trust
- circumscribed problems involving unrealistic expectations of others

---

People do not live in vacuums – they live with others. Everything they do is affected by the people around them – from earliest development (see Chapters 9 and 10) to their later relationships. It's hard to imagine, then, trying to explain their development without taking into consideration their relationships with others – both in terms of their actual relationships and the way they think about those relationships. Feelings of love and anger, for example, seem inseparable from the people to whom they are directed. That's exactly what many psychoanalysts and psychotherapists after Freud thought, and their ideas formed the basis of what became **object relations theory**. To begin to think about this, let's consider Ms A:

Ms A just reached the bus after running six blocks in high heels. Breathlessly, she reaches into her purse to get her prepaid transportation card and realizes that she left it at home. She only has a $10 bill. Ms A asks the driver if he has change, and he does not. The other passengers stare at her blankly, offering no help. She is enraged and throws her $10 at the driver, curses, and takes her seat. Later that day, Ms A feels ashamed about the morning episode and anxious about who might have seen her behave this way. She realizes that this kind of outburst has sometimes led to bad outcomes, for example, in high school when she had to stay for detention after cursing at a teacher, and recently, when her boyfriend broke up with her after an argument that got out of hand.

Psychodynamic Formulation, First Edition. Deborah L. Cabaniss, Sabrina Cherry, Carolyn J. Douglas, Ruth L. Graver, and Anna R. Schwartz.

Why does Ms A have difficulty managing her temper? She clearly struggles with her anger, and this might be rooted in conflict, but could it be related to expectations stemming from early relationships? Let's first describe this way of thinking about development and then see how it can help us to understand Ms A.

Basics of object relations theory

In the 1940s, a group of analysts including W.R.D. Fairbairn, D.W. Winnicott, Michael Baliant, John Bowlby, and Harry Guntrip developed a set of theories later called **object relations theory**. This theory, which builds on concepts initially developed by Melanie Klein, suggests that early interactions with important caregivers help shape the way we come to think, feel, and behave [54, 55]. These early relationship experiences are **internalized** and exist in the individual's unconscious as he/she grows up. Internalization is the process by which people take in their experiences throughout development and make them part of themselves. Internalization of experience occurs throughout the life cycle and, as people get older, is more often called **identification** [49]. Internalized representations of people's earliest experiences offer basic **templates** for relationships that affect all subsequent experiences.

Children's basic templates are of their relationships with their primary caregivers. In most situations, children develop positive relationship templates when caregivers fulfill their needs and negative relationship templates when their needs are unfulfilled [56]. Children can develop both positive and negative templates about the same caregiver.

Internal relationship 1: need-fulfilling

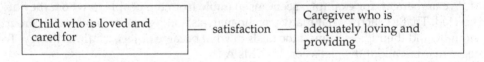

Internal relationship 2: need-frustrating

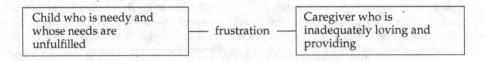

If children are more often satisfied than frustrated in their relationships with early caregivers, they tend to learn to trust others and to develop healthy, balanced expectations of future relationships [57]. On the other hand, if they are predominantly frustrated, children may have difficulty learning to trust others and may develop problematic expectations of future relationships (see Chapter 10). For example, they may come to expect that they will be mistreated or neglected. These expectations, although unconscious, may continue to operate in their adult relationships – even if the situation does not warrant them.

As we have mentioned, children may feel predominantly frustrated by their caregivers either because of the caregivers' limitations or because of a poor match between what the child needs and what the caregiver can offer. For example, a temperamentally difficult-to-satisfy infant may struggle with a well-meaning caregiver. Alternately, a resilient infant may thrive despite a caregiver's limitations.

To explore the way early templates can affect adult relationships, let's return to Ms A, the enraged commuter. Reviewing her history, we learn that when Ms A was 2 years old, her mother became depressed after a miscarriage. Using object relations theory, we can hypothesize that Ms A had unmet needs during this time, producing unconscious anger. Here's how we might depict that template:

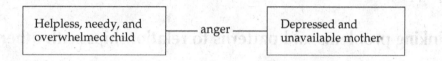

When Ms A is frustrated as an adult – as she was on the bus – she expects that the people around her (like her mother) will be unavailable and unhelpful. This makes her angry and produces behavior that might be more appropriate for a frustrated child than for an adult on a bus. Conceptualizing it in this way helps us to think about how Ms A's early experience with a depressed mother may have influenced her ability to manage disappointment in her current adult life.

For another example, consider the case of Mr B:

> Mr B works for a bank and is responsible for collecting late mortgage payments. His mother was very ill with cancer when he was a young man. He always wished that he had spent more time with her before she died, rather than remaining focused on his social life. He is struggling at his job because he has a hard time collecting payments from people in hardship, especially when medical problems are involved.

Using object relations theory, we can wonder if Mr B's problem collecting mortgage debt is related to an early template of his relationship with his mother, in which he depicts himself as selfish and inattentive. This idea about himself in relation to his mother makes him feel guilty:

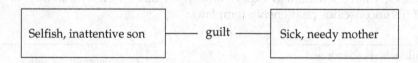

We can then hypothesize that this unconscious template is activated when he has to collect mortgage payments from struggling people – he feels too guilty and is unable to function well in his job. This idea helps us to connect his history to the development of his current problems and patterns.

Relationship patterns are multidimensional

Everyone's unconscious has many of these relationship templates. Most are not problematic and are seamlessly integrated into the way we think about ourselves and others. Templates generally cause problems when they are derived from painful or confusing experiences.

It's also important to remember that people can experience themselves in either role of a relationship template – sometimes they feel like the child and sometimes like the caregiver. This is because, as children, we identify with our caregivers. For example, Mr B, the mortgage collector, might sometimes feel like the selfish child and sometimes like the needy parent. When Mr B has children of his own, he may identify with his mother and feel angry and neglected when his children exhibit age-appropriate selfishness.

Linking problems and patterns to relationships with others

Linking problems and patterns to early unconscious templates is helpful when trying to understand both global and more circumscribed problems with relationships.

Global relationship problems involving lack of trust

Patients who developed problematic early relationship templates often have tremendous difficulty trusting people in their adult lives:

Example

Mr C is a 45-year-old single man who has never had a significant love relationship. He avoids emotional intimacy, works late hours and weekends, and never dates any one person for very long. He recently tried Internet dating and reports, "All women are self-centered – they just want to get pregnant. They view me as a 'sperm machine.'" Mr C's parents divorced when he was 6 years old, leaving him with his mother, who was self-centered, insecure, and determined to find a new husband. He remembers that on many weekend evenings, before going out, she tried on multiple outfits, asked him questions about how flattering they were, and then left him alone for the rest of the evening.

Mr C may have difficulty with intimacy and dependency because his earliest relationships have led him to expect little from others. Here is a way to depict one of his unconscious relationship templates:

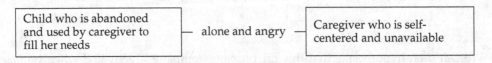

Using object relations theory, we can hypothesize that this unconscious relationship template becomes activated when Mr C meets women, leading him to expect that they will be self-centered and exploitive. This way of linking his difficulties to his early relationship templates helps us to understand Mr C's current problems and to plan therapy.

More circumscribed relationship problems involving unrealistic expectations of others

People who have already attained object constancy (see Chapter 10) and have nuanced views of themselves and other people are less likely to grossly distort interpersonal experiences. Nevertheless, they may still suffer when they have unrealistic expectations of others, which are based on early templates. Object relations theory can be very helpful in understanding these situations, for example, with Ms D:

> Ms D is generally very content with her work and her family life and tends to be a stable, reliable partner to her husband. When her father-in-law developed a terminal illness, her husband became preoccupied and unavailable. As the months wore on, Ms D felt angry with her husband but was unable to express these feelings because, as she said, "they're understandable." Ms D has a younger sister who had childhood leukemia and required a lot of parental attention and long trips away from home to get treatments. Ms D recalled with pride that she was praised for being so independent, well behaved, and "grown up."

Ms D has a well-integrated sense of herself and her important early caregivers. However, although she has attained object constancy, during the period of her sister's illness she may have developed a relationship template related to the expectation that she behave like an adult:

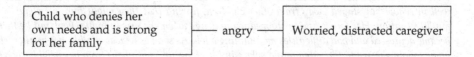

This template, including the feeling of anger toward her parents, remained unconscious and Ms D remained aware only of her wish to help her family. Now, in her adult life, the similarity of the situation activates this unconscious template, causing her to be angry with her husband as if he were one of her distracted parents. Using relationship templates, we can make the link between the unconscious feelings Ms D had as a child and her current difficulties with her husband. This may offer her the opportunity to see that just because her husband is caring for his father does not mean that he will neglect her. It may also help her to alter her expectations of others in her adult life.

A sample formulation – linking to relationships with others

Formulating with object relations theory means explaining problems and patterns by tracing them back to early relationships. Here's an example:

Presentation

Ms E is a 29-year-old woman who presents with difficulty in her relationship with her boyfriend of 6 months. She says that he threatened to break up with her after finding out that she had had sex with a male coworker. "I don't even know why I did it" she says, "But after a few months, I always start to feel dissatisfied with the guy I'm with." She says that this also happens in jobs, and she has had as many as 10 jobs in the past 2 years. She says that the timing is "ironic" because she and her boyfriend had just started to talk about moving in together. "I don't think that he's really in it for the long haul – guys never are." She has few friends and, in the first session, asks if the therapist gives out her home phone number. "My last shrink didn't – what was I supposed to do at midnight after a fight?"

DESCRIBE the problem and patterns (*focused*)

*Ms E has **difficulties in relationships** with others. She does not **trust** others, and she creates situations in which others cannot trust her. Her relationships are **not secure**, and she frequently ruptures them prematurely. These patterns are global in that they affect her romantic relationships, her friendships, and her work situations.*

REVIEW the developmental history

Ms E is the younger of two children born to two active heroin users. Her mother died when Ms E was 2 years old, leaving her in the care of her father. She says that she is not sure whether her mother was abusing drugs while she was pregnant. Her brother, who is 4 years older, corroborates that the two children were left alone – often overnight – when Ms E was as young as 3 years old. She depended on her brother but says that he was "wild" and that, beginning when she was about 6 years old, her brother would occasionally get into bed with her and touch her breasts. Ms E did well in school but stayed away from other children, fearing that they might find out about her family situation. Her father finally stopped using drugs when she was in high school, but he then became depressed and had difficulties maintaining a job. As soon as he was eligible, her brother left home to join the army. She often found solace in "hooking up" with boys from her neighborhood, "I knew that they didn't really care, but it felt good to be next to someone." She ultimately finished college and became a social worker to "try to help kids who grew up the way I did," but she has drifted from placement to placement, generally due to interpersonal difficulties with her coworkers.

LINK the history and problems/patterns to relationships with others

Ms E's difficulties with relationships may be related to her difficulty with her childhood relationships. Given her parents' active drug use, it is likely that Ms E was poorly cared for from birth. Her subsequent history is filled with abandonment (mother's premature death, father's frequent absences, brother's leaving for the army), as well as neglect and abuse.

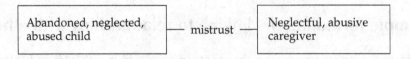

Ms E may have an early template in which she expects to be abandoned and abused by people with whom she has relationships. Consequently, she has not learned to trust others. In order to survive, she has not allowed herself to trust other people, including her romantic partners, friends, and people with whom she works. The closer she comes to imagining that she could trust someone, the more anxious she becomes. This prompts her to create situations in which the relationship is ruptured.

Linking to relationships with others guides treatment

Linking problems and patterns to early relationships suggests that our work should involve helping people to understand their problematic templates and to develop new, healthier ones. As we discussed in Chapter 10, children who suffer from abuse and neglect have trouble achieving object constancy and may persist in splitting in order to maintain positive images of problematic early caregivers. Object relations theory suggests that people will reactivate their early relationship templates with the therapist in the **transference**, which can be interpreted and understood. As people become more aware of their negative relationship templates in therapy, they often improve their ability to tolerate more ambivalent connections to people. Over time, they can develop more complex, nuanced images of important early caregivers. As this occurs, the need for splitting decreases and object constancy improves [58].

In addition to insight, psychodynamic psychotherapy provides a new relationship – the relationship with the therapist. This new relationship can provide the basis for new, healthier relationship templates. For example, patients who are used to having distracted parents may experience a new type of relationship with an attentive therapist [59]. Here is an example of how this technique can work:

Ms F is a 30-year-old publicist who, as a child, was yelled at and punished when she didn't follow instructions. She tried to be perfect and lived in fear of triggering a disciplinary reaction from her parents. In high school, if a teacher was critical of her homework, Ms F trembled – as if she were a helpless child about to be punished. In college, Ms F was anxious, checking things multiple times, and unable to sleep before exams. Now, at work, she still cannot relax and has anxiety attacks before quarterly reviews, thinking that she is about to be fired.

An important relationship pattern for Ms F may be of an abusive, critical authority figure and an imperfect, vulnerable child. These two images are connected by an affect – fear. Ms F internalized this relationship template and alternately identifies herself as either a frightened child or an aggressive authority:

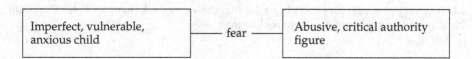

This fundamental template may be activated when relationships resonate with any of these components, even if they are not exactly the same as her early experience. Thus, Ms F felt this at school with her teachers, in college, and now at work with her boss. Here's how this could be addressed in treatment:

> In therapy, Ms F was always careful to get everything right in sessions and seemed anxious if she forgot to pay a bill on time or arrived a few minutes late to a session. Her therapist, Dr Z, noticed this and commented to Ms F that she expected him to get angry with her for these minor issues. Over time, Ms F realized that she had an expectation of Dr Z that was based on an early relationship template – she was behaving as if Dr Z were a punitive, abusive authority figure. Ms F then realized that she was also having the same reaction to her boss. This insight enabled her to rethink whether her boss was really critical or whether she was just experiencing him as if he were a parent and she were still a helpless child. She began to understand that their adult work relationship had room for healthy criticism. She began to experiment with communicating to her boss how she felt about his critiques and became able to discuss with him which points she thought were warranted and which ones were not. In addition, she learned how to negotiate with the therapist to rearrange her session times when necessary and to relax when she needed to pay her bills a few days late.

These interactions led to the internalization of new relationship templates for Ms F, ones populated by more understanding authorities. In object relations theory, the new experience with the therapist is a large part of what is therapeutic.

Suggested activity

What relationship templates might be operating in these people?

> Ms A is a 51-year-old single woman who is "always there" for her friends. She'll babysit for their children, pick up groceries for them, and spend endless hours on the phone with them listening to them complain about their husbands. Recently, she had a colonoscopy. When she arrived, the receptionist asked who would be available to take her home. "No one," she said, "They are all busy. I'll take a cab."

> Mr B is a 45-year-old man who takes his wife out to an expensive restaurant for her birthday. They are shown to a table that is next to the restroom. He is noticeably disturbed and asks to see the maître d'. "You probably think that we saved all year to come here," he says, raising his voice. "But our money is the same as theirs. I don't see why we can't sit at a good table."

Comment

Ms A is very available for others but feels that she cannot ask them for help. She could have a relationship template that looks like this:

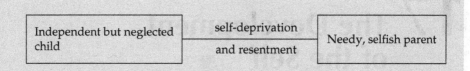

| Independent but neglected child | self-deprivation and resentment | Needy, selfish parent |

Mr B assumes that he is being taken advantage of. He could have a relationship template that looks like this:

| Exploited and unfavored child | — anger — | Self-centered, neglectful parent |

17 The Development of the Self

Key concepts

Self psychology is an organizing idea about development that LINKS problems and patterns to the development of the self.

According to this idea, early caregivers perform functions that are essential for the child's development of the self. These are called **selfobject functions** because they are experienced by the child as part of the self. They are listed below:

- **Mirroring** – the caregiver's empathic ability to appropriately reflect the child's abilities and internal states
- **Idealization** – the caregiver's ability to be idealized by the child

Linking problems and patterns to the development of the self is particularly helpful when constructing case formulations for patients who have problems with

- self-esteem regulation
- empathy and envy

For centuries, philosophers have pondered the question of how to define the self. We think of the self as the essential attributes of a person that are relatively stable over time and that make a person unique. Having a coherent sense of who we are, how we feel about ourselves, and our likes, dislikes, abilities, and limitations is essential for healthy psychological functioning. So is a generally positive sense of self-esteem, characterized by an acceptance of our positive and negative qualities and the capacity to maintain good feelings about ourselves in a variety of contexts, including adversity or criticism from others (see Chapter 4).

The development of healthy self-esteem is thought to depend both on inborn characteristics, such as resilience and optimism, and on relationships with early caregivers. How caregivers respond to their children's emotional states and developing physical and cognitive abilities plays a crucial role in helping children to feel good about themselves and to have a positive but realistic sense of their capacities and

Psychodynamic Formulation, First Edition. Deborah L. Cabaniss, Sabrina Cherry, Carolyn J. Douglas, Ruth L. Graver, and Anna R. Schwartz.
© 2013 John Wiley & Sons, Ltd. Published 2013 by John Wiley & Sons, Ltd.

limitations. Heinz Kohut, a psychoanalyst who was active in Chicago in the 1960s and 1970s, developed a theory of psychological development that focused on this emerging sense of self and that came to be known as **self psychology**. This chapter focuses on this organizing idea about development and the way that we can use it in creating psychodynamic formulations.

Basics of self psychology

As with object relations theory, self psychology focuses on the way early relationships impact development, in particular, the way in which parenting fosters the development of a coherent and vital sense of self. The center of this idea is that the development of the self depends on empathic caregiving. An empathic caregiver is able to accurately sense what a child is thinking and feeling, to show the child that he/she understands this, and to respond to the child in an affectively attuned and developmentally appropriate manner. This is called **mirroring**. Children also need to be able to **idealize** their caregivers – they can then bask in the glow of that idealization in order to feel strong, good, and safe. In addition to mirroring and idealization, self psychology suggests that **grandiosity** in childhood is essential for the development of healthy self-esteem and that this has to be allowed and encouraged by caregivers [53, 60, 61]. Grandiosity includes intense feelings, such as being powerful, special, or beautiful. Empathic caregivers acknowledge and reflect these feelings back to the child in age-appropriate ways.

Kohut coined the term **selfobject** [53, 60, 61] to describe these critical caregiver functions. The word is not hyphenated, which reflects the way in which he believed young children experience their caregivers as not completely separate from themselves. Selfobjects, such as parents or other caregivers, allow themselves to be used by their children to regulate their self-esteem and emotional states.

Example

A 3-year-old girl is playing "house" with her mother. She tells her mother to play the role of the little girl while she plays the mother and instructs her mother very specifically about everything she is to do and say. The mother complies cheerfully, and in her role as "baby," tells the "mother" how nice and pretty she is. The little girl, imitating her mother's voice, says, "I'm the best mommy in the world."

In this example, the mother responds empathically to her daughter's age-appropriate wishes to play with, idealize, and control her. The little girl's identification with her mother, whom she feels is "the best," makes her feel strong and powerful and helps her to build her own sense of self. In addition, the mother's mirroring of the pride her daughter feels helps the little girl to develop self-esteem.

Conversely, children who grow up with caregivers who are preoccupied or distracted, or who are psychologically unable to empathize with the emotional states and needs of their young children, may have trouble developing healthy self-esteem. Similarly, children with caregivers who fail to help them understand their limitations may grow up to have an unrealistically grandiose sense of self that is overly vulnerable to the ordinary slings and arrows of life.

Example

A 5-year-old boy runs into the house, yelling that he is a superhero who has just beaten the villains in a game of tag. He bumps into a table and knocks a vase full of flowers onto the ground, spattering water and bits of pottery everywhere. His father storms into the room, yelling, "Look at the mess you made! Why can't you watch where you're going? Some superhero you are – if you have special powers, let me see you put that vase back together again! I thought so, you can't do it."

In this example, the father does not respond empathically either to his son's need to feel joyful, powerful, and special (playing the role of a superhero) or to the developmentally common occurrence of knocking something over by accident. He is angry with his son and treats him in a humiliating way, teasing him about not having special powers. We can hypothesize that if the father typically treats his son this way, the boy may be at risk for not being able to feel adequately strong and powerful.

Example

A 9-year-old girl auditions for the school musical. Although she has never performed before, or taken singing or acting lessons, her parents tell her, "You're the best singer and actress in the whole school, and if they don't cast you in the lead role they're idiots." One of her classmates, who has been studying singing and acting for several years, gets the lead part. The girl, sobbing, tells her parents how unfair it all is. Her parents say, "You should quit the play, that director is incompetent. We'll call the principal to complain."

In this example, the parents communicate unrealistic expectations to their daughter. When she does not meet them, they blame the director rather than helping her to understand the role that experience and practice play in achievement. In this way, they hinder her ability to assess her capabilities and limitations in a more realistic way. We can hypothesize that this girl is at risk for developing a falsely elevated sense of self, which may crumble in the face of frustrations, leading to rage and externalization of blame.

Both of these examples are isolated incidents – even the most empathic and patient caregivers will occasionally get frustrated or lose their temper. Situations like these are likely to have pervasive and enduring effects only if they represent frequent and typical ways in which caregivers interact with their children. In fact, self psychology asserts that all caregivers will, at some point, fail to respond empathically to their children but that this failure is actually necessary for development. When this failure happens, in an age-appropriate and not exaggerated way, children learn to **internalize their caregivers' selfobject function**. This is important in helping them to learn to buoy their self-esteem and to assess their capabilities and limitations realistically.

Linking problems and patterns to the development of the self

Linking to the development of the self is most helpful when trying to understand problems related to self-esteem. In addition, difficulty in interpersonal relationships stemming from problems with empathy for or envy of others can be well understood using this idea about development.

Self-esteem regulation

Low self-esteem

Low self-esteem can be usefully understood using self psychology. Adults whose earliest caregivers did not recognize and acknowledge their abilities (mirroring) may underestimate their capacities and have difficulty feeling good about themselves. Such people may present for therapy with problems related to underachievement and difficulty in their interactions with others, such as being exquisitely sensitive to criticism, feeling easily blamed or attacked, or tending to castigate themselves. They are also often particularly prone to shame.

Example

Ms A is a 40-year-old woman who comes to treatment complaining of chronic low-grade depression and feelings of low self-esteem. She lives alone, has no children, has never been married, and works as a veterinary assistant. She was reportedly diagnosed with a learning disability in her early teens but never received any sort of help or treatment for it. She explains, "My parents just told me to work harder, like they had." Ms A is attractive and personable, but describes herself as "stupid" and "a loser." She says, "I always thought I'd get married and have a family, but the relationships I've been in have never worked out. I guess when guys really get to know me, they realize that I'm messed up – why would they want to be with me?" When the therapist gently points out how self-critical Ms A is, she says, "I guess that's just one more thing that I can't do right." Ms A felt that her parents were too busy worrying about her two older brothers, or caught up in their own problems, to pay much attention to her. Since her father died a few years ago, Ms A has spent a great deal of time visiting and helping her mother, who she describes as constantly critical.

Ms A's "critical," "distracted" parents may not have given her the mirroring she needed to develop a strong sense of self. Her report that her parents' remedy for her learning disability was simply an edict to "work harder" suggests that they were not attuned to her realistic capacities and limitations. Using self psychology, we might formulate that these empathic failures and lack of appropriate mirroring have resulted in Ms A's inability to have positive feelings about herself.

Overly inflated, but fragile, self-esteem

As we've discussed, mirroring can be problematic if it underestimates *or* if it overestimates a child's abilities. People whose early caregivers overestimated their abilities may have a false sense of self that is outwardly overly inflated but actually extremely fragile. These people may seek help because they, like their caregivers, overestimate their abilities and then have trouble tolerating the disappointment of not attaining their goals. Although they may present as overly confident or arrogant, in the face of self-esteem threats they may quickly become anxious, enraged, or devastated. Patients with this type of problem may seek out others to bolster their self-esteem, and thus their relationships often seem shallow and manipulative. They may become easily discouraged when they can't achieve as much or perform as well as they believe they should.

Example

Mr B is a 33-year-old lawyer. He was recently passed over for promotion, while a colleague who started at the firm when he did was just made partner. Mr B was referred to therapy by his internist whom Mr B consulted, complaining of "heart palpitations." No cardiac abnormalities were found. Mr B reports that he feels anxious and angry much of the time. He says that he is thinking of leaving his firm because the partners are "obviously idiots for thinking that guy [who made partner] is better than I am. He didn't go to an Ivy League school like I did and he's such a dork." He hopes that one of his friends, another lawyer whose family is "incredibly well connected," will land him a job in a prestigious firm. Mr B tells the therapist, "My internist is one of the best doctors in the city – I only go to the best – so if he recommended you then you must be tops."

When the therapist takes a history, he learns that Mr B is an only child whose father is a wealthy and influential businessman in his hometown. He describes his mother as a "social climber" and says that both parents were very focused on his academic and athletic achievements, showering him with praise when he did well and contempt when he did not. Using self psychology, we could formulate that his parents' overemphasis on success prevented Mr B from developing a realistic sense of himself and a healthy sense of self-esteem. Instead, he developed a fragile sense of self that is overly reliant on superficial markers of success and exquisitely vulnerable to self-esteem threats.

Problems with empathy and envy

Children who fail to form a strong sense of self can grow up to have little capacity for empathy and tremendous envy of others. As adults, they are often preoccupied with protecting their own fragile sense of self and are not attuned to the needs, experiences, or perspectives of others. This can be a chronic problem, or can be acute during periods of stress, such as medical illness or emotional distress. As we've discussed (see Chapters 4 and 5), this can lead to problems in relationships with others. Consider Ms C:

Ms C is a 30-year-old woman with a 1-year-old daughter. She comes to therapy with the complaint that "having a child ruined my life." Ms C says she no longer has any time to herself to relax, exercise, or socialize. She feels frustrated with and angry at her daughter much of the time, feeling that she is "too needy" and "spoiled." She doesn't understand how her friends with children have the patience to sit and play with them. Ms C describes her own mother as "really narcissistic," noting that her mother rarely displayed much interest or pride in her.

Self psychology might suggest that growing up with inadequate mirroring, Ms C developed a brittle, fragile sense of self. This limits her ability to think about the needs of others, including her child. Needing to offer empathic mirroring to her own child, when she herself was deprived of this, may be particularly difficult.

Envy can also be well understood using ideas about the development of the self. People who have a balanced but generally positive sense of themselves can tolerate the idea that others have things that they lack. However, people who struggle with maintaining their self-esteem are often threatened by what others have – possessions, abilities, or relationships. Envy (see Chapter 4) can be aggressive and destructive and can make it difficult to have relationships with others.

Example

Mr D is a 24-year-old graduate student who is working in a lab. Despite hard work, his investigations are slow moving and have not engendered much excitement at lab meetings. When his colleague's experiments result in an important discovery, he is publicly derisive of the colleague's results and starts rumors that the colleague "has no ideas of his own – his mentor does all the work." Mr D's father left the family when he was age 5, and he was raised by his mother. He was aware that his father had remarried and lived with his new wife and two children, although he did not see him for many years. When he did see him as a teenager, his father bragged about his new family and told Mr D that he should "take a tip on how to behave from your half-brothers."

Abandoned by his father, and later harshly compared to his father's new "favored" children, Mr D was likely unable to develop a stable sense of self. It is reasonable to imagine that he had nearly intolerable envy of the new children who had usurped his place with his father. Now, as an adult, he is similarly unable to tolerate the success of his "lab sibling," and his envy leads him to be aggressive in an effort to destroy his colleague's success.

A sample formulation – linking to the development of the self

Presentation

Mr E is a 35-year-old high-school history teacher. He is anxious at work much of the time, feeling as if he is always "performing" for his students. Although he gets good evaluations from students and faculty, he struggles with not feeling good, smart, or funny enough. Although he believes that being a teacher is a "noble" profession, he wishes that he had a higher paying, more prestigious job, and he is intensely envious of his friends and acquaintances who do. In his spare time, he plays guitar and harbors secret fantasies of forming a rock band and becoming famous.

DESCRIBE the problem and patterns (*focused*)

*Mr E has frequent symptoms of anxiety and chronic feelings **of low self-esteem** and **envy** of others. He is not able to experience satisfaction at work despite a belief in the value of his job and evidence that he does it well.*

REVIEW the developmental history

Mr E is the youngest of three children whose parents divorced when he was 2 years old. He describes his father, who had been in the military, as frequently depressed, and his mother as irritable and preoccupied. He remembers often feeling lonely as a child. His older sisters were outstanding students and very popular, and he felt that he always lived in their shadow. His mother effusively praised him when he did well in school or at sports, but he felt that "she wasn't really interested in who I was as a person." He did not spend a lot of time with his father in childhood, but remembers trying to "cheer him up" by singing or making jokes, which his father either ignored or reacted to "in a lukewarm way." He also remembers that when, at age 6, he told his father that he wanted to be in the army, his father said, "Don't waste your life like I did."

LINK the history and problems/patterns to the development of the self

Using self psychology, we can postulate that Mr E did not have adequate selfobjects in childhood; his parents were not empathically attuned to him and he was not able to idealize them. Consequently, he was unable to develop a healthy sense of self. His efforts to idealize or enliven his father were met with dismissal or lack of response. He felt outdone by his older sisters, and his mother seemed uninterested in his inner life, while excessively praising his achievements. As an adult, he is unable to take appropriate pleasure or pride in himself and his work, feels chronically anxious about how he appears to others, and takes refuge in fantasies about unattainable goals.

Linking to the development of the self guides treatment

Linking problems and patterns to the development of the self suggests that the therapist's therapeutic strategy should be to help the patient to develop a healthier sense of self. In self psychology, this is thought to happen via the therapeutic relationship itself. Patients look to the therapist to serve selfobject functions, that is, to help stabilize, restore, or enliven their sense of self. Such patients tend to treat therapists not as separate, independent people, but as extensions of themselves over whom they expect to have control. This signals a reactivation of a developmental process that was never fully or optimally completed in childhood. Essentially, these patients use the therapist to satisfy their unmet developmental needs to idealize and gain affirmation and validation of their experiences, states of mind, and grandiose sense of self. They want and need to experience the therapist as all-powerful, special, or perfect. Thinking self psychologically, this kind of idealization is seen not as a defense but rather as an important phase of the treatment, intended to help shore up a shaky sense of self.

Thus, rather than interpreting these transferences early on, the therapist allows them to flourish. Under the influence of these selfobject transferences, the patient can feel understood and enlivened and can experience feelings of union with or control over the therapist. Inevitably, however, the therapist will not always respond just as the patient desires, and these **empathic failures** may cause the patient to feel frustrated or angry. If the empathic failure is appropriately timed and not too intense, the therapist can point it out and discuss it with the patient, who can then start to see the therapist as a separate, flawed, but nevertheless good and caring person. Hopefully, patients can then begin to offer themselves what they have needed and desired the therapist to do for them – affirm their feelings of specialness and power, comfort them, and validate their experiences.

Example

Mr F is a 55year-old electrician who has become a weekend triathlete. He spends his sessions regaling his male therapist with tales of his athletic prowess – passing others in the last moments of races, "shocking" younger competitors by telling them how old he is, and having female racers "come on to him." His therapist listens, hypothesizing that Mr F, who reports that his parents were "disappointed" that his "learning disability" precluded him from going to a prestigious college like his siblings, needs to demonstrate his abilities to a new, idealized man. After Mr F wins a triathalon that he was particularly excited about, he becomes angry that the therapist "didn't seem very excited about it." He spends several sessions telling his therapist that although he "thought" that he was interested in him, he now sees that he was wrong. The therapist acknowledges how disappointed Mr F is in him. After his next big win, Mr F notices that although the therapist may not be giving him the kind of excited reaction he hoped for, he is interested and attentive. Over time, Mr F realizes that he is able to feel good enough about himself without the fantasied reaction from the therapist.

The therapist's steady, empathic attunement to the patient, and his interpretation of the perceived empathic failure, helps Mr F to internalize the mirroring function he craved. This helps Mr F to buoy his sense of self gradually without the continuous congratulations of others, as well as to have a more measured expectation of the people around him. This technique helps people to develop a healthier sense of self that is more resilient in the face of self-esteem threats.

Suggested activity

How might you link the difficulties of these people to problems with the development of the self?

Mr A gets a big bonus at work and comes home with a bottle of wine to celebrate with his wife. She, however, has her hands full with the children and has had a long day – she greets the news with, "great honey – can you run to the store and get some more milk?" He becomes depressed and has fantasies of seducing his administrative assistant, who he thinks has a crush on him.

Ms B invites her coworkers over for a dinner party. For weeks in advance, she discusses her menu – everyone is looking forward to the meal. When they arrive, she is disorganized and prepares a fairly simple dinner of chicken and vegetables. She is enraged when people leave early and are not complimentary.

Comment

When he does not receive immediate kudos from his wife, Mr A is deflated and has fantasies about being admired by his assistant. This suggests that he has a continued need for mirroring from a selfobject and that without it he cannot maintain his self-esteem.

Ms B misperceives her abilities to cook and entertain, and then is angry when others do not share her self-assessment. This suggests that she received problematic mirroring as a child – perhaps her talents were overestimated by parents who needed to see her as more capable than she actually was.

18 Attachment

Key concepts

Our last organizing idea about development, called **attachment theory**, LINKS problems and patterns to early attachment styles.

According to this idea, early attachment styles affect how people develop their sense of self, relationships with others, ways of adapting to stress, and patterns of self-regulation.

Adult attachment styles are categorized as either secure or insecure. There are three types of insecure attachments – avoidant, ambivalent, and disorganized.

Adult attachment styles are thought to be the product of the child's temperament, the parents' attachment pattern and temperament, the interaction between parent and child, and the environment.

Linking to early attachment styles is particularly useful when constructing case formulations for patients who have problems with

- self-regulation, including self-control and affect regulation
- empathy and mentalization

Two women, Ms A and Ms B, go for job interviews. After each interview, the prospective employer gives an equivocal smile and says, "Thank you for coming in. We'll be in touch." Ms A shakes off her residual nervous energy by walking around the block, then goes home, tells her roommate about the interview, watches TV, and goes to sleep. Ms B, however, is undone by the interview and its ambiguous end. She tries to fight the impulse to call the interviewer but fails, texting her to ask whether she should send more references. She calls her roommate and reviews the interview many times, incessantly asking, "What do you think? Do you think I'll get it?" She eats a pint of ice cream and later has two drinks before she tries to sleep, which she is unable to do. Both women endured a stressful situation that left them in limbo, but while Ms A was able to regulate herself after the experience, Ms B was not. Why?

One way to think about this is that Ms A has developed the ability to self-regulate as a result of having developed secure attachments, while Ms B's inability to soothe herself has resulted from her insecure attachment style. As we discussed in Chapter 10, an enormous amount of development happens in the context of the child's dyadic relationship with the primary caregiver. This relationship mediates the development of fundamental capacities that allow the person to begin to have a sense

Psychodynamic Formulation, First Edition. Deborah L. Cabaniss, Sabrina Cherry, Carolyn J. Douglas, Ruth L. Graver, and Anna R. Schwartz.
© 2013 John Wiley & Sons, Ltd. Published 2013 by John Wiley & Sons, Ltd.

of self, form relationships with others, adapt to stress and anxiety, and self-regulate. The style with which infants attach to their primary caregivers has been shown to carry over into the way they attach to others as adults. By describing adult attachment styles, **attachment theory** helps us to understand early relationships and how they contribute to the development of a person's problems and patterns.

Basics of attachment theory

Attachment theory starts with the idea that people are born with a predisposition to become attached to caregivers in their earliest years [62, 63]. The sense of safety that children get from their central caregiving relationship helps them to develop the system of emotional regulation that they use to handle a wide variety of experiences. This experience of nurturance and protection is encoded in the brain and, over time, helps people to develop both the ability to predict and understand their environment and a psychological sense of security [64]. In addition, these interactions help them to develop relatively stable patterns of adapting to stress and regulating their responses to anxiety and affects [65].

As we discussed in Chapter 10, these early patterns of connection, which are called **attachment styles**, are classified as either **secure** or **insecure** and are relatively stable after the first year of life [66]. Children who have secure attachments tolerate separations well and are easily soothed by their primary caregivers when reunited with them, while children who have insecure attachments become highly anxious during separations and are not easily soothed after reuniting [67, 68]. These attachment styles have been shown to predict the comfort with which children experience their environments later in development and carry over to the way they adapt to stressful situations as adults. In other words, the style of attachment that children have by age 1 may be a major contributor to the way they develop their ability to regulate their reactions to stress, anxiety, and affect, and is likely to predict the way they will respond to their internal and external environments as adults [69].

Categories of attachment in adults

To review, the attachment styles of young children are described as either secure or insecure:

- secure
- insecure – has three subcategories:
  - avoidant
  - ambivalent
  - disorganized

These styles correspond to children's behavior at age 1 when observed in brief separations from the mother (see Chapter 10) [64, 67]. Not surprisingly, when adults are interviewed about how they cope with stress and anxiety, specifically in regard to intimate relationships, their attachment styles fall into four similar categories [70, 71]. These adult attachment styles include the way people recall and describe early childhood relationships (particularly those that had significant negative aspects) and the way they describe their current relationships with others. These are the adult attachment styles [72–74]:

Secure

People with this adult attachment style easily remember experiences of others, are able to incorporate painful memories into their discussions, can think about others in three-dimensional terms, and can look at emotions from other people's point of view. They find it relatively easy to become emotionally close to others and are comfortable both depending on others and having others depend on them.

Insecure

There are three subcategories of insecure attachment in adults:

Dismissive/avoidant

This attachment style is characterized by rigid, overly regulated affect. People with this style dismiss attachment as being of minimal value or importance and remember little of their childhood bonds. They may also offer idealized portraits of people in their lives. When probed, however, they are often able to remember incidents suggesting parental neglect or rejection. These people present as strong and independent but are in actuality unable to face the reality of early disappointments.

Preoccupied/anxious

In contrast, people with this attachment style hold themselves responsible for problems in their relationships and idealize their early caregivers. They are anxious and worried about relationships with others and about how they are perceived. They often find it hard to speak in an organized way about their past relationships. They are consciously preoccupied with their early caregivers and remain very reliant on them. In their adult relationships, they seek high levels of intimacy and are often very dependent.

Disorganized

This is the most disturbed adult attachment style. People with this attachment style often have dramatic fluctuations in their descriptions of others and may be unable to recall past relationships. Many people with this attachment style have a history of trauma or loss of a parent and have a high chance of repeating trauma with their own children. Their adult relationships are fairly chaotic; for example, they typically enter quickly into intense relationships and then become easily mistrustful and withdraw.

For example, consider the differences between Mr C's and Mr D's attachment patterns:

> Mr C comes to therapy because he has been anxious since his daughter went away to college. His history reveals that he was an anxious child. He remembers screaming at the chain-link fence in the playground when his mother left him at elementary school. In adolescence, he became despondent after a girlfriend broke up with him. When he talks about his daughter, he speaks haltingly and starts to tear up, saying "I don't know why she couldn't have gone to college closer to home. How could she do this to me?"

> Mr D comes to therapy because his wife is complaining that he overworks and will not curtail his work life to spend time with his family. Their daughter told his wife that she wishes she had a closer relationship with him. Mr D reports this with little concern and, staring out the window, says, "She's doing fine. I think a daughter's primary relationship is with her mother."

In these examples, Mr C has a **preoccupied/anxious** pattern of attachment, while Mr D's attachment pattern is **dismissive/avoidant**.

Attachment styles are passed on from parent to child

People with each adult attachment style tend to have children with a related attachment style. This process is referred to as **intergenerational transmission of attachment** (Table 18.1).

Empathy and the development of affect regulation

Why does one adult have one attachment style vs. another? Children are more likely to develop adaptive, secure attachment styles if their caregivers can understand and process their emotional experiences (this is also called mentalization, see Chapters 6 and 10) [78, 79]. The caregivers' processing of emotion fosters the development of the child's ability to **regulate affect**, that is, the ability to handle basic emotions, such as fear, anxiety, insecurity, and excitement [80, 81]. When the caregiver is unable to empathize and respond sensitively, however, children are likely to develop insecure attachments that predispose them to chronic difficulty with self-regulation, particularly related to modulating their sense of self, their capacity for impulse control, and their reaction to anxiety [82, 83].

Table 18.1 Intergenerational transmission of attachment [75–77]

Caregiver's adult attachment style	Child's attachment style
Secure →	Secure
Insecure: dismissive/avoidant →	Insecure: avoidant
Insecure: preoccupied/anxious →	Insecure: ambivalent
Insecure: disorganized →	Insecure: disorganized

Linking problems and patterns to attachment styles

Attachment theory helps us to formulate in cases in which self-regulation and affect regulation are impaired, as they often are in people with insecure attachment. It can also be helpful in understanding patients who have difficulties with empathy and mentalization, which contribute to problems with interpersonal relationships.

Problems with self-regulation and managing affect

Self-regulation and managing affect can be difficult for people with insecure attachment styles. This is often evident around challenges such as loss, separations, and life transitions. Dealing with divorce, freshman year of college blues, changing jobs, managing illness, and losing a loved one are just a few of the many separations and losses that highlight problematic attachment patterns and bring people to psychotherapy.

Example

Mr E and F started dating in medical school. When they started separate medical internships at different institutions, Mr E became very anxious – but adapted by staying in regular contact with F via text messages. As the months of the internship unfolded, Mr E became more panicked and clingy. One day, F could not respond to a text because she was conducting a procedure. Mr E panicked and called 911 to find her. In therapy, Mr E reported that his father died when he was young and his mother coped with her grief and anxiety by staying in almost constant contact with him.

Using attachment theory, we can hypothesize that Mr E developed his anxious attachment style in response to his mother's preoccupied/anxious attachment style. This insecure style of attachment impaired his ability to regulate affect and anxiety and has led him to have an insecure attachment to his girlfriend. In therapy, he realized that his difficulties were connected to his early relationship with his mother and he learned that there were other ways to manage his anxieties about separations from F.

Difficulty with empathy

Attachment theory is also helpful in understanding patients who have difficulty with empathy. Consider the following example:

When Mr G hears that his wife has planned an evening out with a friend, he becomes enraged, accusing her of no longer wanting to spend time with him. As a child, Mr G's father presumed that he was "guilty until proven innocent" and routinely punished Mr G without asking him his side of the story.

Taught by his father, Mr G is unable to imagine what his wife might be thinking when she decides to spend time with a friend. Instead, he assumes that she is thinking what he is thinking. He is also unable to empathize with her wish to socialize with others.

Parenting is another situation in which empathy is essential, as in the following example:

> Ms H is a single mother whose 5-year-old daughter has been having great difficulty staying in school without her mother. She is referred for psychotherapy by the school psychologist. Ms H explains that her daughter has few friends, keeps to herself, and sits at the sidelines while the other children play. Ms H says, "I've been dealing with my sick mother and haven't been around much lately. She seems to manage fine, though; she hardly complains." Ms H tells the therapist that her daughter suffers from asthma and was hospitalized several times as a baby. When the therapist asks Ms H about her own childhood, she learns that Ms H was also a withdrawn child.

Using attachment theory, we could suggest that Ms H's dismissive attitude toward her daughter is related to her avoidant attachment style, now emerging in her daughter as well. Offering Ms H other perspectives – for example, that perhaps her daughter is reacting to the early hospitalization, as well as to worry about her grandmother's illness – allows Ms H to understand her daughter's experience. Ms H can then process her daughter's feelings and help her daughter to do this as well. This will help both Ms H and her daughter to gain more access to their feelings.

A sample formulation – linking to attachment

Presentation

> Mr I has become increasingly distraught since his daughter, who previously lived down the block with her husband, announced she was getting divorced. Mr I and his wife are very upset that their daughter will be moving into an apartment further away. Although he says that he knows that he's overreacting, he talks quickly and loudly in therapy and asks if he can have a "double session" because he has so much he needs to talk about.

DESCRIBE the problem and patterns (*focused*)

> Mr I has profoundly **insecure** relationships. He reacts strongly to change and to loss. His family has long felt that he smothers them. He didn't allow his children to go more than a car ride away to college and doesn't understand why this bothers them. He thinks his daughter should work things out with her husband who he thinks is "a terrific guy" but who never worked and who is fully supported by his daughter.

REVIEW the developmental history

> Mr I grew up in a tightly knit family with an anxious mother who currently lives with him and his wife. He recalls having few friends as a child and being kept home by his mother to watch TV with her. His father, who passed away several years before, was a WWII veteran who had been injured and had fairly severe PTSD. His only brother moved away years before and was estranged from the

family after numerous disappointments related to his not coming home for family events/holidays. Mr I did well in school and had opportunities to pursue college away from home but chose a modest community college so that he could continue to live with his parents. He married young – his wife, who is also anxious, has become devoted to his mother as well.

LINK the history and problems/patterns to attachment styles

Mr I's pattern of becoming increasingly anxious and demanding in the face of disappointment and loss may be indicative of his anxious/preoccupied attachment pattern, which is also present in his mother. Mr I tries to draw people closer (his daughter, the therapist) in order to decrease his own anxiety, but, in so doing, he inadvertently pushes them away (the daughter feels misunderstood; the therapist has no choice but to end the session). This makes him more anxious. He also has difficulty imagining other peoples' internal experiences (mentalization), perhaps because his overwhelming desire to preserve the attachment connection prevents him from considering any needs other than his own.

Linking to attachment styles guides treatment

In psychotherapy, patients repeat their attachment styles with their therapists. Together, patient and therapist can then observe and identify the attachment style. This can facilitate change in two ways – by making people aware of their attachment patterns and by helping them to attach in new ways.

Becoming aware of attachment styles

Becoming more aware of their characteristic attachment styles and how they evolved enables patients to create new narratives about themselves [84]. Consider the following example:

Ms J had always blamed herself for being an oversensitive, chronically anxious child. In therapy, she learned that the death of her mother's father and her parents' long-term marital difficulties had made her mother anxious during most of her childhood. She realized that her own anxiety was a reaction to her mother's anxious state. Having a new understanding about the origin of her anxiety helped her to feel more relaxed and increased her empathy for her mother.

Ms J has a preoccupied/anxious attachment style. With a new way of thinking about her life story, Ms J is more able to accept both her own anxiety and her mother's.

Improving affect management

People with a disorganized attachment style can have difficulty with affect regulation, especially during periods of intense emotionality. When this occurs within a therapy session, the therapist can help the patient to manage his/her feelings by describing what is happening and by helping the patient to think about what might be happening in the minds of both the patient and the therapist [85]. To illustrate this, consider Ms K, who has a disorganized attachment style:

> Ms K began telling her therapist, Dr Z, about her history of sexual abuse just as the session was ending. She became more confused and lost track of time. Dr Z stated, "This is a hard subject to discuss, particularly when there are only 5 minutes left to the session." Ms K became enraged that Dr Z was ending the session abruptly, saying, "You don't care about me ... I'm not sure I ever want to come back here." Dr Z commented, "I see how talking about the abuse disorients you, so much that you feel that I, too, am against you. Can you imagine any other ways of looking at what just happened between us?" This helped Ms K to calm down and to consider that Dr Z's interruption may have sounded abrupt, but in fact reflected her worry about the patient.

Using attachment theory, Dr Z thought about Ms K's outburst as the result of her attachment style. She empathized with Ms K's experience and realized that Ms K was unable to consider that Dr Z had an alternate reason to end the session in that way. By asking her to consider other ways of looking at the situation, Dr Z was helping Ms K to manage her feeling of being hurt by the therapist. Repeating this in therapy can help the patient to process intense feelings more effectively in situations outside of the treatment as well [86].

Developing a more secure attachment style

Over time, patients can change their attachment styles as they develop a more secure attachment to their therapists. This is thought to occur as therapists repeatedly experience, observe, and describe the way their patients handle feelings. Patients internalize this, gradually learning to have a clearer and more flexible idea of what goes on in their minds and in the minds of their therapists. In the context of a more secure attachment, patients can develop functions that they were not able to develop as children, such as an increased ability to self-regulate and to modulate affects. Let's consider an example of someone with a dismissive/avoidant attachment style who has difficulty experiencing affect:

> Ms L is a 52-year-old gay woman who lives apart from her long-term partner. Her partner complains that Ms L is emotionally distant and removed. After 20 years together, they recently got married and Ms L says she's tired of putting up so many walls. In treatment, Dr Y notices that Ms L speaks hesitantly in sessions and often becomes quiet and looks away after he speaks. When Dr Y inquires about this, Ms L reveals that she is afraid that he doesn't approve of her. She then talks about how harshly critical her mother was. Ms L then begins to consider that perhaps Dr Y is trying to be helpful and begins to speak more freely.

Of particular note is the way Ms L's attachment style is communicated nonverbally – she turns away. Therapists using techniques from attachment theory are attuned to the nonverbal as well as verbal ways of understanding their patients' attachment patterns. Over time, observing and describing these patterns in the relationship with the therapist allows patients to feel secure enough to consider alternative ways of managing their feelings.

Suggested activity

How would you describe the attachment styles of these adults?

Ms A is a 40-year-old woman who married her high-school classmate. When her husband suggests that they attend their 25th college reunion, she says, "Why would I want to do that? Just to see a lot of middle-aged losers? I'd rather go to the gym."

Mr B, a 21-year-old college student, had a tumultuous relationship with C that ended in a breakup. When he sees C in the bookstore after summer vacation, he has the sensation that he is going to throw up, leaves his books in the middle of the aisle, and runs in the opposite direction.

Comment

Ms A likely has a **dismissive/avoidant** attachment pattern. Although she remembers past relationships, she does not value them and has a rigid, overly independent stance.

In contrast, Mr B's behavior suggests a **disorganized** attachment pattern. When he sees his ex-girlfriend, he behaves in a bizarre manner.

Putting it Together – A Psychodynamic Formulation

Now that you've learned to DESCRIBE, REVIEW, and LINK, let's listen in as one therapist, Dr Z, puts together a psychodynamic formulation. Dr Z has seen his patient, Mr C, for four evaluation sessions. We'll hear some of Dr Z's thought processes as he

- hears the presentation
- DESCRIBES the problems and patterns after asking questions about the patient's general functioning
- REVIEWS the developmental history
- LINKS the problems and patterns to the history by
  - focusing what he's learned from DESCRIBING and REVIEWING
  - asking a focus question
  - choosing ideas about organization
- writes a chronological narrative
- thinks about how his formulation will guide his treatment

Let's start with Mr C's presentation:

Presentation

Mr C is a 28-year-old graphic designer who presents to the clinic saying that he is depressed after a "huge fight" with D, his girlfriend of 6 months. Mr C says that he and D had been having difficulty for the last few weeks, precipitated by his feeling that she no longer wanted to be in a relationship with him because she wanted some "time to herself." Mr C says he became "terrified" that D would leave him and began texting and calling her at all hours to "make sure" that she still loved him. Three days ago, while they were arguing at D's apartment, C says that he "refused to leave" until he had D's "guarantee" that they would stay together. He finally left after D threatened to call the police. Since then, he has felt "frantic," has not gone to work, has barely gotten out of bed, and has had very little appetite. He made the call to the clinic after a coworker texted him and suggested that he talk to someone about the situation.

> After hearing the presentation, Dr Z thinks:
>
> *"The thing that really jumps out at me is how terrified Mr C was that his girlfriend might leave him. That's what led him to react so dramatically. I wonder how he functions in other aspects of his life?"*
>
> Dr Z then goes on to ask Mr C about other aspects of his general functioning. Here's what he DESCRIBES:

DESCRIBE

Problem

Mr C has had several days of oversleeping, poor appetite, and inability to get out of bed after a tumultuous fight with his girlfriend. These symptoms were not present prior to this episode. The couple has had several weeks of arguing prompted by Mr C's fear that his girlfriend would leave him.

Patterns

Self

*Mr C has strengths and difficulties in this area. He believes that he is a good designer and seems to have reasonable **self-perceptions** about his work and creative abilities that are neither grandiose nor self-deprecating. At work, he is generally able to handle **self-esteem threats**, such as having others critique his work, without becoming overly emotional. In his romantic relationships, however, he often responds to self-esteem threats related to rejection with tremendous anxiety and fear.*

Relationships

*Mr C's personal relationships tend to be **insecure**, marked by **lack of trust**, rapid but shallow **intimacy** followed by estrangement, a **poor sense of self and other** with **lack of empathy**, and fear of abandonment. This is particularly true in his romantic relationships. For example, the pressure of his need to be reassured by D prevented him from taking into consideration her feelings, or from considering her way of perceiving the situation.*

Adapting

*Mr C uses different **defenses** in different situations. At work, he uses more adaptive defenses, such as humor and excessive emotionality. In his personal relationships, however, he tends to use **less adaptive defenses**, such as splitting, projection, idealization, and acting out. His style of adapting tends to **emphasize emotions** and to be **inflexible**. Again, in the context of his personal relationships, he has difficulty with **managing his emotions** – as was evident from his behavior with D, he is unable to "sit with" his anxiety. Although this leads him to be **impulsive** with his girlfriend (e.g., constant calling and texting), he does not have difficulty controlling his impulses with substances or at work. He does not report difficulty with **sensory regulation**.*

Cognition

Mr C graduated with high marks from a prestigious design school. He has been praised for his ability as a graphic designer, and he has also scored well on his high-school standardized tests. Thus, he seems to have talent and is likely to be **intelligent**. At work, he collaborates with a team and is able to **solve problems** and to be **creative**. In his romantic relationships, however, he has great difficulty **mentalizing** and is not particularly **self-reflective**.

Work and play

Mr C **supports** himself as a graphic designer. He works hard and has difficulty relaxing on weekends and holidays. He has few friends and tends to spend his **leisure time** cloistered with the woman with whom he is currently involved.

After several evaluation sessions with Mr C, Dr Z begins to focus what he has DESCRIBED:

"Mr C's greatest difficulties seem to be with insecure relationships and managing emotions. Since he has the most difficulty managing emotions in the context of relationships, I'm going to focus on RELATIONSHIPS. Here's the question I'd really like to answer in my psychodynamic formulation:

Mr C seems very intelligent, talented, and creative, but he has such anxiety about his relationships he ends up destroying them. Why is that?"

Dr Z then learns about Mr C's developmental history:

REVIEW

Genetics and prenatal development

Mr C is the youngest of three children born to married parents. He denies that there were any prenatal exposures or birth injuries, and he was a term baby born at 7 pounds. Mr C says that his mother likely had untreated anxiety her whole life – he says she's a "nervous wreck" who thought that everything was a "catastrophe." He does not believe that his mother was physically ill during her pregnancy with him or that she used substances during that time. He thinks that other members of his mother's family might have anxiety as well. He does not know his father or his father's family well enough to give this history. He also says that his mother has always said that he was a difficult baby, who cried a lot, did not want to be left alone, and was "clingy."

Earliest years (birth to age 3)

Although Mr C says that he has few memories from this time, his older brothers have told him that his parents were "constantly fighting." He has vague memories of his father slamming doors and of his mother crying on the couch. Mr C says that any memories of these years are generally of his brothers excluding him, and he feels that he spent much of his time alone. Mr C's father, a businessman, left his mother when Mr C was 3 years old and quickly started a new family with a *woman with whom he had been having an affair for most of his short marriage. He moved across the country, and although he continued to send occasional checks, he had little direct contact with Mr C and his older brothers. His earliest memory is of his mother screaming at him on a street corner – he thinks that it was because he had momentarily let go of her hand and she was afraid that he might be hit by a car.*

Middle childhood (age 3–6)

After his father left, Mr C says he and his mother became much closer. He developed nightmares and could only sleep if his mother was with him. Mr C says, "My brother teased me mercilessly, saying I was a baby. I wanted to be able to sleep alone, but I couldn't do it." At around age 6, his mother started dating a coworker and abruptly insisted that Mr C sleep in his own bed when the boyfriend began to sleep over. Mr C says, "It still makes me upset, practically like it's happening right now." He had trouble separating every year at the beginning of school – in kindergarten, his mother had to sit in the "coffee room" for weeks – long after all of the other children were just being dropped off. Although he was embarrassed about this, he remembers feeling "panicked" at the thought of being in school without her.

Later childhood (age 6–12)

Mr C says he was lonely during later childhood. He had one or two male friends and says, "We read a lot of comics but we didn't really talk to each other much." Home life was stressful – his mother remained in an on-again, off-again relationship with the boyfriend who was a heavy drinker. He says, "The one thing I remember that was good was that I started drawing; it began with making comics like the ones we read, and I was good at it." When at home, his mother was anxious, forcing him to wear overly warm clothing and fretting about his homework, but she would frequently forget to pick him up from school and occasionally spent the night with her boyfriend without letting her children know.

Adolescence (age 13–18)

Mr C began to be noticed in school for his unusual drawing and math skills. A teacher encouraged him to apply for a scholarship to a local summer art program that he attended for several years and he ultimately won a nationally recognized prize. He says, "Thank goodness for that; it saved me." He reports he had sex for the first time, "younger than most kids; I was probably about 15. I was the kind of kid who always had a girlfriend but they never lasted very long." He experimented with marijuana and cocaine but found that they made him feel uncomfortable and did not continue to use them. He drank fairly heavily during a relationship with a girl who liked alcohol, but stopped when they broke up. Once his brothers had moved out of the house, he rarely saw them; he avoided his mother who had started to drink heavily and was rarely home overnight.

Young adulthood (age 18–23)

Mr C was accepted into a prestigious design school in his home city. Although he had planned to live with his mother, within a few weeks of matriculation he had met and moved in with his first "serious" girlfriend. He felt that he had met his "soul mate," but within a few months they were fighting. Throughout his design school years, Mr C had serial relationships with women that began "like gangbusters" and then ended tumultuously. Mr C did very well in school, won many awards and prizes, and was offered several good jobs on graduation.

Later adulthood (age 23 to present)

Mr C now supports himself and feels comfortable at his workplace. He is interested in starting his own firm but fears breaking away from his current colleagues. His longest relationship lasted almost one year and ended when his girlfriend told him that she was gay. He was "devastated," but quickly began to date D.

Now Dr Z tries to focus what he has REVIEWED:

"I think that the most problematic parts of Mr C's history occurred during his earliest years and middle childhood. They also involve relationships – particularly his overly close but inconsistent relationship with his mother early in life, and the fact that his father basically abandoned him at age 3."

Dr Z now tries to LINK Mr C's problems and patterns to his developmental history: *"So, from DESCRIBE, Mr C's greatest difficulty is his lack of secure relationships – he needs to be so close to his girlfriends that he ends up emotionally strangling them. From REVIEW, the most problematic part of Mr C's history is his overly close but inconsistent relationship with his mother, as well as the fact that his father abandoned him. Insecure relationships generally result from problems like these. This makes me think that I could use ideas about attachment to LINK his patterns to his history. But, you know, Mr C was apparently anxious from birth, and his mother has anxiety as well – this could be a temperamental trait. So I should factor in ideas about the impact of early cognitive and emotional difficulties as well – they may be important on their own and in the way that they shaped his early attachments. He also has important strengths that developed during later childhood and adolescence that are helping him to function in important ways – I need to include that, too. I'll focus on the early development of his attachment problems, and then try to see how that affected his development throughout his life."*

LINK

Mr C's area of greatest difficulty is his relationships with others. This is most likely related to his insecure (preoccupied/anxious) style of attachment, which leads him to become frantic and emotionally dysregulated when he fears abandonment. This scenario led to his current presentation and has occurred many times in the past. Mr C's insecure attachment style has its origin in his earliest relationships.

Temperamentally anxious and fearful of separation, Mr C spent his earliest years in an environment filled with violent parental disputes. He experienced his mother as tremendously anxious, frequently tearful, and preoccupied. Thus, it is likely that he had difficulty establishing a solid dyadic relationship. Frequently alone and afraid, he never developed basic trust or the capacity for a secure attachment. His mother's anxiety and preoccupation suggests that she was not particularly attuned to Mr C – he thus had difficulty developing a sense of his own affect states, or those of others. This has likely contributed to his adult difficulties with empathy, mentalization, self-regulation, and trust.

Thus, Mr C entered middle childhood with an insecure attachment and without having consolidated many crucial capacities. His developmental trajectory was further hindered by the fact that his father had recently left home – he remained locked in his two-person relationship which his mother sexualized by bringing him into bed with her. In the absence of a rival, this is likely to have overwhelmed him and exacerbated fears of losing this all-important relationship. It also fueled aggression from his older brothers, surrogate rivals who further terrified him. His mother's abrupt expulsion of Mr C from her bed and his replacement by a new boyfriend may have crushed and confused him. This oscillation between inappropriate closeness and abrupt abandonment likely led to his anxious attachment style.

The inconsistency in his relationship with his mother continued into later childhood. Either his mother was overly concerned about his attire or she was forgetting to pick him up from school. His school-age separation anxiety may have been related to his temperamental anxiety, but may also have been related to his developing insecure-anxious attachment style. It is likely that his mother's problematic relationship with her alcoholic boyfriend, as well as her own increased drinking, worsened her inconsistency and, consequently, Mr C's attachment problems.

In school, Mr C's difficulty with same-sex peer friendships may have resulted from many factors, including his lack of a male role model to help him to feel like a strong boy, and his temperamental anxiety. His sense of self was weak because of his problematic dyadic relationship and the absence of his father, and was buoyed a bit by his discovery of drawing, which gave him pleasure as well as attention. This talent, the mentorship of his teachers, and his artistic successes are the features of his developmental history that helped him most and that are most responsible for the self-esteem that he derives from his work.

Mr C's precocious sexual relationships were most likely attempts to regain the security of his lost dyadic relationship. They set the stage for the series of intense, short-lived relationships that have characterized his young adulthood. The continuation of his insecure attachment style as a young adult has rendered him virtually unable to be alone, leading him to emotionally strangle his partners and to, time after time, destroy the very relationships to which he desperately clings.

This formulation led Dr Z to think that Mr C would only alter his insecure attachment style in the context of the therapeutic relationship. He therefore recommended twice weekly psychodynamic psychotherapy. He wondered how his formulation would change as the treatment progressed …

Suggested activity

Now it's time to write a complete psychodynamic formulation of your own. Focus what you've DESCRIBED and REVIEWED, and then select organizing ideas about development that you think will usefully LINK them to form hypotheses about causation. Begin with a summary, and then try to trace the development of the person's major difficulties and strengths throughout his/her life. Don't forget that you can use many organizing ideas about development in a single formulation. Once again, try to share your work with a peer or a supervisor – talking about the choices you made in constructing your formulation will enhance your learning.

Part Four References

1. van der Kolk BA, McFarlance AC. The black hole of trauma. In: van der Kolk BA, McFarlane AC, Weisaeth L (eds.). *Traumatic Stress: The Effects of Overwhelming Experience on Mind, Body, and Society*. Guilford Press: New York, 2007: 3–23.

2. Herman JL. *Trauma and Recovery: The Aftermath of Violence from Domestic Abuse to Political Terror*. Basic Books: New York, 1992.

3. American Psychiatric Association. *Diagnostic and Statistical Manual of Mental Disorders*, 4th edn. American Psychiatric Association: Washington, DC, 1994.

4. Breuer J, Freud S. On the psychical mechanism of hysterical phenomena: Preliminary communication. In: Strachey J. (ed.) *The Standard Edition of the Complete Psychological Works of Sigmund Freud (1893-1895): Studies on Hysteria, Volume II*, Hogarth Press: London, 1893: 1–17.

5. Carlson V, Cicchetti D, Barnett D *et al*. Disorganized/disoriented attachment relationships in maltreated infants. *Developmental Psychology* 1989; **25**: 525–531.

6. Cicchetti, D, Toth S. A developmental psychology perspective on child abuse and neglect. *Journal of the American Academy of Child and Adolescent Psychiatry* 1995; **34**: 541–565.

7. Edwards V, Holden G, Felitti V *et al*. Relationship between multiple forms of childhood maltreatment and adult mental health in community respondents: Results from the adverse childhood experiences study. *American Journal of Psychiatry* 2003; **160**: 1453–1460.

8. MacMillan H, Fleming J, Streiner D *et al*. Childhood abuse and lifetime psychopathology in a community sample. *American Journal of Psychiatry* 2001; **158**: 1878–1883.

9. Paolucci E, Genuis M, Violato C. A meta-analysis of the published research on the effects of child sexual abuse. *The Journal of Psychology* 2001; **135** (1): 17–36.

10. Stovall-McClough KC, Cloitre M. Unresolved attachment, PTSD, and dissociation in women with childhood abuse histories. *Journal of Consulting and Clinical Psychology* 2006; **74** (2): 219–228.

11. Bremner JD, Randall P, Vermetten E *et al*. MRI-based measurements of hippocampal volume in posttraumatic stress disorder related to childhood physical and sexual abuse: A preliminary report. *Biological Psychiatry* 1997; **41**: 23–32.

12. Heim C, Nemeroff CB. The impact of early adverse experiences on brain systems involved in the pathophysiology of anxiety and affective disorders. *Biological Psychiatry* 1999; **46**: 1509–1522.

13. Teicher M. Wounds that time won't heal: The neurobiology of child abuse. *Cerebrum* 2000; **2** (4): 50–67.

14. Teicher MH, Andersen SL, Polcari A *et al*. The neurobiological consequences of early stress and childhood maltreatment. *Neuroscience Biobehavioral Review* 2003; **27**: 33–44.

15. Stein MB. Hippocampal volume in women victimized by childhood sexual abuse. *Psychological Medicine* 1997; **27**: 951–959.

16. Yehuda R. Biology of posttraumatic stress disorder. *Journal of Clinical Psychiatry* 2001; **62** Suppl 17: 41–46.

17. Bremner JD. Long-term effects of childhood abuse on brain and neurobiology. *Child and Adolescent Psychiatric Clinics of North America* 2003; **12**: 271–292.

18. Hofer MA. On the nature and consequences of early loss. *Psychosomatic Medicine* 1996; **58**: 570–581.

19. McFarlane A, de Girolamo G. The nature of traumatic stressors and the epidemiology of posttraumatic reactions. In: van der Kolk, B, McFarlane A, Weisaeth L (eds.). *Traumatic Stress: The Effects of Overwhelming Experience on Mind, Body, and Society*. Guilford Press: New York, 2007: 129–154.

20. Yehuda R. *Psychological Trauma*. American Psychiatric Publishing, Inc.: Washington, DC, 1998.

21. McFarlane A, Yehuda R. Resilience, vulnerability and the course of posttraumatic reactions. In: van der Kolk BA, McFarlane AC, Weisaeth L (eds.). *Traumatic Stress: The Effects of Overwhelming Experience on Mind, Body, and Society*. Guilford Press: New York, 2007: 155–181.

22. Foa E, Stein D, McFarlane A. Symptomatology and psychopathology of mental health problems after disaster. *Journal of Clinical Psychiatry* 2006; **67** (Suppl 2): 15–25.

23. van der Kolk BA, Roth S, Pelcovitz D *et al*. Disorders of extreme stress: The empirical foundation of a complex adaptation to trauma. *Journal of Traumatic Stress* 2005; **18**: 389–339.

24. Kilborne B. When trauma strikes the soul: Shame, splitting, and psychic pain. *American Journal of Psychoanalysis* 1999; **59**: 385–402.

25. Lansky, MR. Shame dynamics in the psychotherapy of the patient with PTSD. *Journal of the American Academy of Psychoanalysis and Dynamic Psychiatry* 2000; **29**: 133–146.

26. Boulanger G. Wounded by reality: The collapse of the self in adult onset trauma. *Contemporary Psychoanalysis* 2002; **38**: 45–76.

27. Fink K. Magnitude of trauma and personality change. *International Journal of Psychoanalysis* 2003; **84**: 985–995.

28. van der Kolk B. The complexity of adaptation to trauma: Self-regulation, stimulus discrimination, and characterological development. In: van der Kolk BA, McFarlane AC, Weisaeth L (eds.). *Traumatic Stress: The Effects of Overwhelming Experience on Mind, Body, and Society*. Guilford Press: New York, 2007: 182–213.

29. Briere J, Gil E. Self-mutilation in clinical and general population samples: Prevalence, correlates and functions. *American Journal of Orthopsychiatry* 1998; **68** (4): 609–620.

30. Briere J. Dissociative symptoms and trauma exposure: Specificity, affect dysregulation, and posttraumatic stress. *Journal of Nervous and Mental Disorders* 2006; **194** (2): 78–82.

31. Briere J, Runtz O. Symptomatology associated with childhood sexual victimization in a non-clinical sample. *Child Abuse & Neglect* 1998; **12**: 51–59.

32. Costello EJ, Mustillo S, Erkanli A *et al*. Prevalence and development of psychiatric disorders in childhood and adolescence. *Archives of General Psychiatry* 2003; **60**: 837–844.

33. Arcelus J, Vostanis P. Psychiatric comorbidity in children and adolescents. *Current Opinion in Psychiatry* 2005; **18** (4): 429–434.

34. Mineka S, Watson D, Clark LA. Comorbidity of anxiety and unipolar mood disorders. *Annual Review Psychology* 1998; **49**: 377–412.

35. National Institute of Mental Health. Mental Illness Exacts Heavy Toll, Beginning in Youth. NIMH Press Release, June 06, 2005. *www.nimh.nih.gov/science-news/2005/mental-illness-exacts-heavy-toll-beginning-in-youth.shtml/* (accessed 12 December 2012).

36. Kessler RC, Berglund P, Demler O *et al*. Lifetime prevalence and age-of-onset distributions of DSM-IV disorders in the National Comorbidity Survey Replication. *Archives of General Psychiatry* 2005; **62** (6): 593–602.

37. President's New Freedom Commission on Mental Health. Achieving the Promise: Transforming Mental Health Care in America. Pub no SMA-03-3832. Rockville, MD, 2003.

38. Kim-Cohen J, Caspi A, Moffitt TE *et al*. Prior juvenile diagnoses in adults with mental disorder: Developmental follow-back of a prospective-longitudinal cohort. *Archives of General Psychiatry* 2003; **60** (7): 709–717.

39. Hyson D. Understanding adaptation to work in adulthood: A contextual developmental approach. *Advances in Life Course Research* 2002; **7**: 93–110.

40. Collins WA, van Dulmen MC. The significance of middle childhood peer competence for work relationships in early adulthood. In: Huston AE, Ripke MN (eds.). *Developmental Contexts in Middle Childhood: Bridges to Adolescence and Adulthood*. Cambridge University Press: New York, 2006: 23–40.

41. The National Advisory Mental Health Council Workgroup on Child and Adolescent Mental Health Intervention Development and Deployment. Blueprint for Change: Research on Child and Adolescent Mental Health, 2001.

42. Giedd JN, Keshavan M, Paus T. Why do many psychiatric disorders emerge during adolescence? *National Review of Neuroscience* 2008; **9** (12): 947–957.

43. Douaud G, Mackay C, Andersson J *et al.* Schizophrenia delays and alters maturation of the brain in adolescence. *Brain: A Journal of Neurology* 2009; **132**: 2437–2448.

44. Jessor R. Successful adolescent development among youth in high-risk settings. *American Psychologist* 1993; **48**: 117–126.

45. Aneshensel CS, Sucoff CA. The neighborhood context of adolescent mental health. *Journal of Health and Social Behavior* 1996; **37** (4): 293–310.

46. Rutter M. Psychosocial influences: Critiques, findings, and research needs. *Development and Psychopathology* 2000; **12** (3): 375–405.

47. Rutter M. Environmentally mediated risks for psychopathology: Research strategies and findings. *Journal of the American Academy of Child and Adolescent Psychiatry* 2005; **44** (1): 3–18.

48. Sroufe AL, Duggal S, Weinfield N *et al.* Relationships, development, and psychopathology. In: Sameroff AJ, Lewis M, Miller SM (eds.). *Handbook of Developmental Psychopathology* (2nd edn). Kluwer Academic/Plenum Publishers: New York, 2000.

49. Moore BE, Fine BD (eds.). *Psychoanalytic Terms and Concepts.* Yale University Press: New Haven, 1990.

50. Cabaniss DL, Cherry S, Douglas CJ *et al. Psychodynamic Psychotherapy: A Clinical Manual.* Wiley-Blackwell: Oxford, 2011.

51. Kris AO. Unconscious processes. In: Gabbard GO, Litowitz BE, Williams P (eds.). *Textbook of Psychoanalysis.* American Psychiatric Publishing, Inc.: Washington, DC, 2012: 53.

52. Freud S. The ego and the id. In: Strachey J. (ed.) *The Standard Edition of the Complete Psychological Works of Sigmund Freud, Volume XIX.* Hogarth Press: London, 1923: 1–66.

53. Mitchell SA, Black MJ. *Freud and Beyond.* Basic Books: New York, 1995.

54. Fonagy P, Target M. *Psychoanalytic Theories: Perspectives from Developmental Psychology.* Brunner-Routledge: New York, 2003.

55. Kernberg O. Psychoanalytic object relations theories. In: Moore BE, Fine BD (eds.). *Psychoanalysis the Major Concepts.* Yale University Press: New Haven, 1995: 450–462.

56. Kernberg O. *Aggression in Personality Disorders and Perversions.* Yale University Press: New Haven, 1992.

57. Winnicot D. Transitional objects and transitional phenomena. *International Journal of Psychoanalysis* 1953; **34**: 89–97.

58. Caligor E, Kernberg O, Clarkin J. *Handbook of Dynamic Psychotherapy for Higher Level Personality Pathology.* American Psychiatric Publishing, Inc.: Washington, DC, 2007.

59. Loewald HW. On the therapeutic action of psychoanalysis. In: Loewald HW (ed). *The Essential Loewald Collected Papers and Monographs.* University Publishing Group: Maryland, 2000: 221–256.

60. Kohut H. *The Analysis of the Self.* The University of Chicago Press: Chicago, 1971.

61. Kohut H, Wolf, ES. The disorders of the self and their treatment: An outline. *International Journal of Psychoanalysis* 1978; **59**: 413–425.

62. Bowlby J. The nature of the child's tie to his mother. *International Journal of Psychoanalysis* 1958; **39**: 350–373.

63. Slade A. The development and organization of attachment: Implications for psychoanalysis. *Journal of the American Psychoanalytic Association* 2000; **48**: 1147–1174.

64. Main M. Discourse, prediction, and recent studies in attachment: Implications for psychoanalysis. *Journal of the American Psychoanalytic Association* 1993; **41S**: 209–244.

65. Fonagy P, Target M. Early intervention and the development of self-regulation. *Psychoanalytic Inquiry* 2002; **22**: 307–335.

66. Ainsworth MDS, Blehar MC, Waters E *et al. Patterns of Attachment: A Psychological Study of the Strange Situation.* Lawrence Erlbaum. Hillsdale, NJ, 1978.

67. Hesse E, Main M. Disorganized infant, child, and adult attachment. *Journal of the American Psychoanalytic Association* 2000; **48**: 1097–1127.
68. Main M. The organized categories of infant, child, and adult attachment. *Journal of the American Psychoanalytic Association* 2000; **48**: 1055–1095.
69. Dozier M, Chase-Stovall K, Albus KE. Attachment and psychopathology in adulthood. In: Cassidy J, Shaver PR (eds.). *Handbook of Attachment: Theory, Research, and Clinical Applications*, Guilford Press: New York, 1999: 497–519.
70. Fonagy P, Steele M, Moran G *et al.* Measuring the ghost in the nursery: A summary of the main findings of the Anna Freud Centre - University College London Parent-Child Study. *Bulletin of the Anna Freud Centre*, 1991; **14**: 115–131.
71. Hesse E. The adult attachment interview: Historical and current perspectives. In: Cassidy J, Shaver PR (eds.). *Handbook of Attachment, Second Edition: Theory, Research and Clinical Applications*. Guilford Press: New York, 2008: 552–599.
72. Fonagy P. *Attachment Theory and Psychoanalysis*. Other Press: New York, 2001: 36–44.
73. Slade A. A view from attachment theory and research. *Journal of Clinical Psychoanalysis* 1996: **5**: 112–122.
74. Lyons-Ruth K, Block D. The disturbed caregiving system: Relations among childhood trauma, maternal caregiving, and infant affect and attachment. *Infant Mental Health Journal* 1996; **17**: 257–275.
75. Fonagy P, The significance of the development of metacognitive control over mental representations in parenting and infant development. *Journal of Clinical Psychoanalysis* 1996; **5**: 67–86.
76. Beebe B, Lachmann FM, Jaffe J. Mother-infant interaction structures and presymbolic self- and object representations. *Psychoanalytic Dialogues* 1997; **7**: 133–182.
77. Van Ijzendoorn M, Schuengel C, Bakermans-Krnenburg MJ. Disorganized attachment in early childhood: Meta-analysis of precursors, concomitants and sequelae. *Development and Psychopathology* 1999; **11**: 225–249.
78. Coates SW. Having a mind of one's own and holding the other in mind: Commentary on paper by Peter Fonagy and Mary Target. *Psychoanalytic Dialogues* 1998; **8**: 115–148.
79. Bouchard M, Target M, Lecours S *et al.* Mentalization in adult attachment narratives: Reflective functioning, mental states, and affect elaboration compared. *Psychoanalytic Psychology* 2008; **25**: 47–66.
80. Schore AN. Effects of a secure attachment relationship on right brain development, affect regulation, and infant mental health. *Infant Mental Health Journal* 2001; **22**: 7–66.
81. Schore A. *Affect Regulation and the Origin of the Self*. Lawrence Erlbaum: Hillsdale, NJ, 1994.
82. Lyons-Ruth K. The two-person construction of defenses: Disorganized attachment strategies, unintegrated mental states, and hostile/helpless relational processes. *Journal of Infant Child and Adolescent Psychotherapy* 2002; **2**: 107–119.
83. Fonagy P. Attachment and borderline personality disorder. *Journal of the American Psychoanalytic Association* 2000; **48**: 1129–1146.
84. Slade A. The implications of attachment theory and research for adult psychotherapy. In: Cassidy J, Shaver PR (eds.). *Handbook of Attachment, Second Edition: Theory, Research and Clinical Applications*. Guilford Press: New York, 2008: 762–782.
85. Fonagy P, Bateman A. *Psychotherapy for Borderline Personality Disorder: Mentalization-Based Treatment*. Oxford University Press: Oxford, 2004.
86. Fonagy P, Bateman A. Randomized controlled trial of outpatient mentalization-based treatment versus structured clinical management for borderline personality disorder. *American Journal of Psychiatry* 2009; **166**: 1355–1364.

PART FIVE: Psychodynamic Formulations in Clinical Practice

Introduction

Key concepts

We can create and use psychodynamic formulations in many different clinical situations, including

- acute care settings, such as emergency rooms and inpatient units
- psychopharmacologic treatments
- psychodynamic psychotherapy

As we learn about our patients, our psychodynamic formulations change.

Psychodynamic formulations can be useful in all clinical settings

Now that we know how to write psychodynamic formulations, how and when do we use them? Students and clinicians often erroneously assume that psychodynamic formulations are only useful for psychodynamic psychotherapy. Nothing could be further from the truth. Psychodynamic formulations help us to understand how and why people think, feel, and behave the way they do, and thus are helpful in every clinical situation. This includes single encounters in emergency rooms, brief therapies on medical or psychiatric inpatient units, psychopharmacologic treatments, and short- and long-term outpatient psychodynamic psychotherapies. In brief clinical situations, our psychodynamic formulations will be based on more limited information about patients and will generally help us to understand one or two aspects of a person's function, such as what brought him/her to the emergency room now. In long-term treatments, our psychodynamic formulations will be based on more extensive information and will help us to understand the broad sweep of a person's development. Regardless of the clinical situation, formulating psychodynamically helps us to understand the impact and development of our patients' unconscious thoughts and feelings.

Psychodynamic formulations are alive and changing

As we discussed in Part I, constructing an initial formulation is extremely useful for many reasons – it helps us to make a treatment recommendation, set goals, and form a therapeutic strategy. However, staying open to new ways of thinking about how and why a person thinks, feels, and behaves allows us to deepen our formulations throughout our work with patients. Psychodynamic formulations are not static – we constantly revise them as we learn more about people during treatment. This new information comes from both what our patients tell us about their histories and our interactions with them.

Let's consider then how we use psychodynamic formulations in many different clinical situations, beginning with acute care settings.

19 Psychodynamic Formulations in Acute Care Settings

Key concepts

Psychodynamic formulations are useful in all mental health treatment settings. This includes the following acute care settings:

- psychiatric emergency rooms
- psychiatric inpatient units
- medical or surgical services

Acute care settings pose special challenges to psychodynamic formulation because

- the clinician's time with patients is usually limited
- patients may be unable to provide a complete history
- the formulation needs to target the acute problem
- the formulation needs to include the predictable stresses related to the acute care setting itself

Even brief, preliminary psychodynamic formulations help us to

- engage patients
- make sense of their current and long-term problems and patterns
- choose the most salient problems and patterns to address
- predict how patients are likely to respond to help
- plan acute and ongoing treatment

Mr A is a 26-year-old graduate student, living with three friends from college, who presents to the emergency room with recurrent bouts of rapid heart rate and difficulty breathing. He is crying, distraught, and frightened that he is going to die. He implores the medical staff to save him. After evaluating his symptoms, the emergency room physician tells Mr A he is having panic attacks and administers lorazepam. This does little to calm the patient and psychiatry is asked to consult.

Psychodynamic Formulation, First Edition. Deborah L. Cabaniss, Sabrina Cherry, Carolyn J. Douglas, Ruth L. Graver, and Anna R. Schwartz.
© 2013 John Wiley & Sons, Ltd. Published 2013 by John Wiley & Sons, Ltd.

If the evaluation of Mr A's presenting problem stopped here, it might be summarized as follows: "26-year-old man with no prior history of mental health problems or treatment presents with new onset of panic attacks." However, even in the setting of the emergency room, it is important to go beyond the presenting problem to ask, "Why did this particular person with his particular life story develop this particular problem at this particular stage in his life?" [1] Here's what happens when Dr Z, the emergency room psychiatrist, comes to talk to Mr A:

> *After reassuring Mr A that his problem is treatable, Dr Z tells him that panic attacks are sometimes precipitated by stress. He asks Mr A whether he can think of anything that is going on in his life recently that might be stressful for him. "It's sort of mystifying," Mr A responds. "When I finished my dissertation last month, I felt like a huge weight had been taken off my shoulders. My advisor loved it. I felt like anything was possible and I went out celebrating with my girlfriend and roommates." He sighs and adds, "But I don't know if I have what it takes to be an academic. My father says you make peanuts teaching high school Latin and keeps asking how I'm going to support myself and a family with a PhD in classics. Please don't tell him I'm here – he already thinks I'm a total loser."*

The additional information that Dr Z has elicited suggests that Mr A may be suffering from feelings of insecurity and low self-esteem related to his father's failure to acknowledge his accomplishments and encourage his independence. This information helps Dr Z to begin to answer the simple but important question "Why now?" and guides him in planning the best way to alleviate the anxiety that brought Mr A to the emergency room.

> *Dr Z asks Mr A to tell him more about his background. Mr A tells him that he has an older sister who was "born normally." His mother desperately wanted a second child, but after a number of miscarriages decided to adopt a newborn: "I've always had this feeling it was more her decision and my father sort of went along with it to make her happy." Mr A knows nothing about his biological parents or the circumstances of his birth, but does not recall being told about any significant problems in his infancy or childhood. He describes his mother as "wonderful, giving, loving," but no match for his father: "Dad and I are close but he's always been a tough act to follow. I did OK in school but didn't get into the prep school or college that everyone in Dad's family attended. I was a good athlete, especially in squash, but Dad was a nationally ranked player in college. Get the picture?"*

At this point, Dr Z has a wealth of information about Mr A. This will help him to think about why Mr A is having anxiety now and to suggest acute treatment. It will also help him to understand Mr A's ongoing problems and patterns and to engage with him in a discussion about possible ongoing therapy. All of this will go far beyond the lorazepam dose in helping Mr A to understand the way in which he is adapting to his current internal and external environment. Dr Z was able to get this information during a short consultation in the emergency room and to use it to construct this psychodynamic formulation:

Mr A is a 26-year-old graduate student in classics who presents to the emergency room with new onset of panic disorder. His panic attacks started in the context of completing his dissertation and beginning to think about future career options. Although he was consciously excited about finishing this work, it is clear that he has been plagued by chronic doubts about his abilities – doubts compounded by his father's tendency to be critical of and to belittle his achievements. He yearns for his father's approval but often feels he has failed to live up to his father's excessively high standards. Thus, conflicts about moving ahead at this point may have triggered anxiety and precipitated the panic attacks. Conflicts between wanting his father's approval and unconscious rage at his father may also have played a role.

Mr A appears to have long-standing difficulties with insecurity and low self-esteem, dating back to childhood. While appropriately proud of his academic successes, Mr A is excessively dependent on his father's opinions, and his view of himself seems to be easily influenced by his father's put-downs. Although he had a close relationship with his mother, it may be that Mr A had difficulty developing a cohesive sense of self because of his father's lack of empathic attunement. He was also an anxious and phobic child, and thus, temperamental factors may also contribute to his difficulties with self-esteem.

Dr Z was able to use this formulation to suggest to Mr A that he was in no physical danger but that he might be having a variety of feelings related to having finished his dissertation. In reassuring tones, he uses this understanding to recommend psychotherapy to Mr A:

Although you're very excited about having finished your dissertation, it sounds like you might be having anxiety about your next steps. Moving forward often comes with anxiety, and that might be helpful to talk about. I think that, in addition to the medication, psychotherapy might be very helpful for you in the coming months.

Thus, even in acute care settings, formulations provide a vital road map for engaging patients, deciding how best to address their difficulties, and predicting how they are likely to respond to our interventions.

Psychodynamic formulations help in all settings

As in the case of Mr A's brief emergency room visit, psychodynamic formulations can help to guide treatment in all clinical situations, including acute care settings. These settings include

- psychiatric emergency rooms [2–7]
- psychiatric inpatient units [8–10]
- medical and surgical services [11–21]

Although we often do not have much time during acute care encounters, we can still form preliminary psychodynamic formulations that help us to understand our patients' unconscious thoughts, wishes, feelings, and fears. Even a preliminary psychodynamic formulation can help us to

- engage our patients
- answer the "Why now?" question
- begin to understand the context of the patient's emotional difficulties
- choose the most important problems and/or patterns to address acutely
- predict how our patients are likely to respond to the help we offer
- plan acute and ongoing treatment

Even if it seems that the immediate crisis is an expectable episode in a chronic psychiatric illness, it is important to ask ourselves whether what is happening could have been triggered by thoughts or feelings that are out of the patient's awareness. Thinking psychodynamically – wherever we are working – guides us to remember that people are often motivated by unconscious thoughts and feelings. Understanding those motivations can be the key to resolving the problems that bring our patients to treatment [5, 18, 21–23].

When formulating in acute care settings, it is useful to remember that these environments affect all patients in somewhat predictable ways [22]. For example, coming to an emergency room often confirms a patient's feelings of worthlessness and failure, while simultaneously activating wishes to be rescued by protective caregivers. Locked inpatient units can stimulate fears of being controlled, while medical and surgical units often trigger fears about death and dying. It is important for us to consider these common reactions when we are trying to understand our patients in acute care settings.

Challenges of psychodynamic formulation in the acute care setting

Constructing psychodynamic formulations in acute care settings presents the clinician with unique challenges. Let's consider a few of them:

The clinician's time with patients is limited

In settings such as an emergency room or an inpatient unit, we generally do not have the luxury of taking a thorough developmental history or waiting for the history to unfold over time. Instead, we often have to rely on information obtained in a single interview to formulate an understanding of the salient problems and patterns and to initiate treatment. Still, even with limited information – gathered from the history as well as from our interactions with the patient – it is possible to develop a deeper understanding of the underlying feelings, fantasies, and fears that may be contributing to the patient's presenting problems. Consider this example:

> *Ms B, a 66-year-old recently widowed woman with long-standing depression, is admitted to the medical service for fever, weight loss, and abdominal pain. Workup reveals chronic myelogenous leukemia, but Ms B refuses further treatment and asks to be discharged, saying, "I've lived long enough." The consulting psychologist, Dr Y, acknowledges the medical intern's concern that Ms B may be "too depressed" to make this life-altering decision but wonders why an otherwise healthy woman would decline treatment that could extend her life for many years. Dr Y explains to Ms B that her medical doctors have asked him to see her because they are puzzled about why she is refusing relatively benign and potentially lifesaving treatment. Ms B responds saying, "What's the point?" and begins to cry. Feeling an unexpected sense of loss, Dr Y says quietly, "It doesn't sound like you feel that there is much reason for going on." Ms B looks at him and nods, saying, "Ever since my husband died 2 years ago, I just haven't been able to pick up the pieces and move on. God knows why – he made my life miserable." Asked to say a little more about her marriage, Ms B says that she was verbally abused and intimidated throughout their 22-year marriage. "Especially when we found out I couldn't have kids, I felt like a failure, like all the mean things he ever said about me were true ... My girlfriends joke that I married my father. He was a mean drunk, too, always raging at my mother over nothing. It was terrifying – sometimes I was worried he'd kill her. When I was a teenager, he up and left with his secretary and I never saw him again."*

While Dr Y may have numerous goals in the consultation, his first priority is to engage the patient by conveying that he hears and recognizes her immediate concerns [11, 12]. When Dr Y echoes Ms B's feelings of futility, she feels understood and shares that she has been depressed since her husband's death, that the marriage was difficult, and that her relationship with her husband recapitulated aspects of her relationship with her father. With these few hints, Dr Y does not continue to probe Ms B's past history, but rather begins to develop an hypothesis that Ms B's treatment refusal may be related to her husband's death. He wonders if resigning herself to dying when she might live a normal life span is related to unconscious guilt about surviving her husband. Dr Y then uses his psychodynamic understanding of the case to try to relieve Ms B's depression and guilt and enable her to accept treatment:

> *Ms B admits that she has been upset with herself for having wished her husband dead at times and says that she feels guilty both about his death and about outliving him. Dr Y suggests that Ms B is blaming herself for something she could not control. Smiling, Dr Y asks Ms B if she could forgive herself for having had one or two aggressive thoughts about her husband, particularly given the verbal abuse she endured for decades. He files away the information about her abandonment by her father but decides to keep the focus on her current feelings of guilt about her husband, which seem more directly relevant to her decision to refuse medical care. After discussing this some more, Ms B ultimately decides to go ahead with treatment.*

Even in a single encounter, Dr Y was able to understand enough about the way Ms B's unconscious guilt may have contributed to her treatment refusal to help her to make more adaptive choices during this stressful time in her life.

The clinician may not be able to obtain a full history from the patient

Patients in acute care settings may be initially unable or unwilling to provide the information needed to formulate a preliminary psychodynamic understanding of their problems and patterns. In this case, it may be necessary to obtain collateral history from relatives, significant others, or outpatient therapists working with the patient and family. It is important, however, to remember that the history obtained from other sources may be affected by their feelings about the patient's situation and thus should be taken with the proverbial "grain of salt."

Example

Mr C, a 47-year-old unmarried man living with his parents, has chronic schizophrenia and has had many prior hospitalizations. He is admitted involuntarily to the psychiatric inpatient unit for an acute exacerbation of psychotic symptoms after flushing all of his medications down the toilet. Although he has often been noncompliant with his medication, the social worker, Mr X, asks himself what prompted Mr C to stop his drugs this particular time. When he asks Mr C why he thinks that he has been admitted to the hospital this time, Mr C glares at him and mutters, "I'm not going to let some terrorist kill my mother." He then turns to the wall and ignores Mr X's questions. Looking frustrated and overwhelmed, Mr C's mother tells Mr X, "My son has never accepted that he needs medication. He's always been stubborn as a mule. Even as a teenager, way before he got sick, he was rebellious and difficult." She says that Mr C's father recently suffered a stroke and adds, "I just don't know if I can handle both of them anymore."

In Mr C's case, Mr X has to rely initially on collateral history obtained from the patient's mother. However, Mr X quickly realizes that the mother's history is colored by chronic anger at her son and decides that taking a more thorough developmental history from her is unlikely to shed much light on Mr C's noncompliance. Nevertheless, he uses the information he obtains to begin to understand Mr C's current issues. For example, he wonders whether Mr C's current episode of noncompliance could be related to fears of losing his father. This understanding helps him to think about ways to reassure the patient that his father is well taken care of – for example, by arranging for home care for the father. Mr X also considers that Mr C's initial hostility toward him could be related to long-standing issues about being controlled by authority figures and begins to think about ways to circumvent this in their next meeting. Although incomplete and gleaned from a family member, the developmental history helps Mr X to construct a brief formulation that will help guide the treatment.

The psychodynamic formulation needs to target the acute problem

Because our work with patients in acute care settings is usually time-limited, the formulations we construct in these settings should target the acute issues. As illustrated in these examples, we always have to ask ourselves, "Why now?" – in other words, is there a specific, circumscribed crisis that led this particular patient to come to the hospital at this particular time? [1] Even after a brief assessment, we can outline the

- **problem** that brought the person to treatment at this time
- **patterns** of thinking, feeling, and behaving that are most directly related to the acute crisis

We can then follow up with a targeted developmental history that explores possible childhood antecedents of these problems and patterns. Although targeted formulations of this kind may feel incomplete, they are vital for helping us to understand our patients and to make choices about treatment.

20 Psychodynamic Formulation in Pharmacologic Treatment

> **Key concepts**
>
> When treating patients with medication, we can use psychodynamic formulations to form hypotheses about problems and patterns that could affect their psychopharmacologic treatment.
>
> In this setting, the most helpful psychodynamic formulations target issues related to
>
> - symptoms
> - medications
> - compliance
> - side effects

Patients who come for mental health care generally seek relief from suffering of some kind. Some may have preferences from the outset about whether or not they want treatment with medication, psychotherapy, or both. Others may not have a particular treatment preference. Increasingly, due to how mental health care is structured, delivered and paid for (at least in the United States), and portrayed in the media, psychiatrists are often called on to "just prescribe medication," leaving the talking out of the cure [24]. Their patients may receive psychotherapy from other mental health professionals, or not at all.

Patients who come for medication visits, however, are just as likely to discuss emotionally meaningful topics as are patients in psychotherapy. The pharmacologists they see need not only to listen and respond empathically to what is troubling their patients [25] but also to realize that this information, when sensitively elicited and understood, often provides crucial insight into the potential effectiveness of the medication in a given clinical situation. The realities of today's psychiatric practice, however, often dictate that psychiatrists limit the time of "med check" visits to 15–20 minutes. Is there a role for psychodynamic formulation in this type of treatment? [26, 27]

Psychodynamic Formulation, First Edition. Deborah L. Cabaniss, Sabrina Cherry, Carolyn J. Douglas, Ruth L. Graver, and Anna R. Schwartz.
© 2013 John Wiley & Sons, Ltd. Published 2013 by John Wiley & Sons, Ltd.

A psychodynamic formulation helps guide pharmacologic treatment

A psychodynamic formulation can be helpful in guiding treatment even when the treatment is envisioned as primarily pharmacologic. Good formulations help clinicians to understand their patient's attitudes toward their illnesses, the prescribing and taking of medication, and the treating clinicians [27].

For the pharmacologist, the most helpful type of psychodynamic formulation is one that is concise and problem-focused. There will be those cases in which the patient has a clear-cut psychiatric diagnosis, few or no comorbid symptoms or conditions, no conflicts about taking medication, good medication response with few or no side effects, and good compliance with the medication regimen. More often, however, the situation is more complex. The patient may have an unclear diagnosis, multiple stressors or traumas, ambivalent or negative feelings about taking medication, troublesome side effects, or difficulty adhering to medication as prescribed. In these cases, the treating clinicians will be well served by taking the time to get to know the patient well enough to construct a targeted psychodynamic formulation. This will also serve to strengthen the therapeutic alliance, which has been shown to correlate positively with treatment adherence and outcome [28, 29]. When a patient is in a **split treatment** (i.e., receiving medication from a physician/pharmacologist and psychotherapy from another clinician), a crucial component of the treatment is the willingness of the clinicians to communicate and collaborate with each other, both in the initial evaluation and in the follow-up phases. This can include exchanging ideas about the psychodynamic formulation.

Gathering information for a targeted formulation in pharmacologic treatment

The way in which a patient presents for the initial consultation will guide the approach to gathering information for the targeted psychodynamic formulation. If a patient presents in a crisis – for example, acutely suicidal – the immediate goal will be to ensure the patient's safety. More extensive history taking can wait. On the contrary, if a patient with long-standing generalized anxiety plans a consultation weeks in advance, we have time to start by getting to know the patient and understanding the "Why now?" of the visit. Of note, some of the data we need for formulation may be obtained by cultivating a good working alliance with the referring clinician, who may be a non-MD psychotherapist or a primary care doctor.

Even in a relatively nonurgent situation, however, there may not be time to take an extensive developmental history, or to explore in depth the patient's current and past relationships. Given the exigencies of the clinical situation, the history taking must be targeted. So, what type of information is useful to know in order to begin to formulate?

Example

Mr A tells Dr Z that he has come for a consultation "because my wife wants me to see you." He says that he's been "a bit depressed, but it's no big deal, I get depressed when work isn't going well." He answers questions reluctantly and offers little information. Gazing at the diplomas on the wall, he says, in a somewhat sarcastic tone of voice, "So, you went to a lot of schools, you must be pretty smart." Dr Z doesn't respond to this, but proceeds to ask a battery of questions regarding Mr A's symptoms.

In this example, Dr Z might conclude that Mr A has five out of nine symptoms of major depression (recurrent, moderate in severity) and may decide to prescribe an antidepressant medication. Mr A's provocative comment about Dr Z's diplomas, however, suggests that other issues may be at play, such as vulnerability to self-esteem threats and difficulty trusting others, which could affect the pharmacologic treatment and his alliance with Dr Z. Without learning more about Mr A, his sense of self, his relationship with others, and his attitudes toward doctors, medication, and psychiatric diagnoses, there's a good chance that the treatment may not be successful [30, 31].

When seeing a new patient for the first pharmacology consultation, it's useful to set the frame by explaining the purpose of the visit. For example:

Although the main goal of today's visit is to see whether or not medication might be helpful to you, in order to best do that I'll have to get to know you as a person. So I'll be asking some questions about your current life situation as well as your past.

The following sections discuss important pieces of information that can help the clinician to construct a targeted psychodynamic formulation for a psychopharmacologic treatment:

A targeted developmental history

In addition to taking a standard medical and psychiatric history, including a history of trauma, it is useful to know something about the patient's childhood and family of origin. This can be woven into standard history taking, by saying, for example,

It would be helpful if you could tell me briefly about yourself and what your family was like when you were growing up. What kind of child were you? What were your parents and siblings like? Is there anything important about your childhood or teenage years that I should know?

In particular, it is important to learn about early temperamental patterns, symptoms of cognitive and emotional difficulties, and medication history – both in the patient and in family members.

History of relationships

A useful way to ask about this is with a question such as

Tell me about the important people in your life.

Try to get the patient to describe them and his/her relationship with them. It can be useful to find out if anyone the patient knows is taking, or has taken, medication for a psychiatric disorder. It is also important to find out upon whom the patient relies for support and who might be a source of stress.

Adapting

Understanding how a patient adapts to stress, self-regulates, regulates sensory stimuli, and manages emotions is invaluable for psychopharmacologic treatment. This can help us to put the concept of medication into a larger context and to suggest nonpharmacologic strategies for managing symptoms. It can also help us to predict a patient's reactions to relapse, side effects, and treatment nonresponsiveness. We can ask the patient

How do you typically manage stress? How do you generally deal with negative emotions such as anxiety, anger, or sadness? How well do you feel those coping strategies work?

Attitudes toward illness

As part of an evaluation, we always take a history of past medical and psychiatric symptoms, disorders, and treatment. In addition to just getting the facts, we can also ask patients about what their experience with illness or treatment has been like, how they understand the current situation or problem, if they have any ideas or theories about what caused or contributed to the current problem, and what they think might be helpful. Questions such as,

Sometimes people have ideas about why they are anxious. Do you?

Or

Even though I know that depression is a medical illness, sometimes people with symptoms like yours worry that they have caused their problems. Have you had any thoughts like that?

Understanding our patients' fantasies about their symptoms can be critical to the success of the treatment.

Attitudes toward medication

There has been a lot of attention given to the topic of psychiatric medication in the media in recent years. It is likely that patients who present to mental health professionals have some preexisting opinions and feelings about medication, and it's important to ask about these when we start the treatment. Patients may know a lot, or little, about psychiatric medications and may have feelings ranging from very negative to quite positive. Often, these attitudes can be elicited by asking whether anyone the patient knows is taking, or has taken, medication for a psychiatric disorder.

Example

Mr B is referred to a psychiatrist by his therapist for evaluation of depression. During the initial interview, Mr B tells the psychiatrist, "My sister has tried several antidepressants and she's had nothing but terrible side effects. I don't have much faith in them."

Also, medication may have specific meanings for patients [31, 32]. Some of these meanings may include a validation that there is something "biological" causing their symptoms, a blow to self-esteem, a "special" form of being taken care of, a means for others (e.g., the psychiatrist) to control their mind or body, and a sense that they have "failed" psychotherapy [32–34].

Example

Ms C's therapist has referred her to Dr Y, a psychiatrist, for consultation about a trial of antianxiety medication. Ms C says, "My therapist really cares about me. She's seen how much I suffer from my panic attacks and wants to do everything possible to make me feel better, so if you and she think that medication will help, I'm ready to try it."

Attitudes toward the treating clinician

Although we usually do not ask patients directly about their attitudes toward us, we look for clues about this and note them during the consultation. Is the patient overly deferential and idealizing? Suspicious and mistrustful? Hostile and argumentative? All of these attitudes signal important information, and the clinician's job is to try to understand their causes and sources. They might indicate symptoms of an underlying psychiatric disorder, or they might be long-standing attitudes that the patient has toward others in a position of authority, for example. These attitudes may certainly have implications for adherence to medication recommendations and effectiveness for any given patient and can help the pharmacologist to take a stance that is most likely to engage the patient [35].

Constructing a psychodynamic formulation in a psychopharmacologic treatment

The psychodynamic formulation in a psychopharmacologic treatment targets the problems and patterns that affect the patient's feelings, attitudes, and behaviors toward medication. In essence, we want to know, "Given this person's problems, patterns of relating to self and others, characteristic ways of adapting to stress and conflict, and significant history, how can I predict how he/she will react to pharmacologic treatment?"

Some of the more common patterns and conflicts that may affect a patient's attitudes toward pharmacologic treatment are problems with self-esteem, trust, and dependency. As mentioned earlier, some patients may feel that receiving a psychiatric diagnosis for which medication is recommended constitutes a blow to self-esteem. The physical fact of ingesting a pill every day can be experienced as a concrete reminder that one is "defective" or is using a "crutch." Patients who have problems with trust may be reluctant to trust the recommendations of a psychiatrist, or to ingest a substance that can cause unpleasant physical sensations or potentially dangerous side effects.

Patients who are reluctant to depend on others may feel that relying on a pill, or on the doctor whom they need to see for the prescription, is a weakness or a blow to their sense of independence or self-reliance. Particularly if a medication is helpful, it can be all the more distressing to anticipate a situation in which it is needed but unavailable. Understanding these common fears can help us to talk to our patients about them and to find strategies for reducing anxiety and increasing therapeutic alliance.

Here are a few psychodynamic formulations constructed in psychopharmacologic treatments. Let's start with this formulation for Mr D:

Presentation

Mr D, a 30-year-old man, comes to Dr X, a psychiatrist, for evaluation of long-standing complaints of anxiety. He has episodic attacks of panic, with shortness of breath and fear that he is having a heart attack, as well as a fear of germs and contamination that lead him to spend long amounts of time each day washing his body, belongings, and apartment. This often makes him late to work and has impeded his ability to have a long-standing romantic relationship. He has come now at the recommendation of his psychotherapist, who feels that a course of CBT can be aided by medication. Despite his distress, Mr D has not wanted to take medication. He describes his symptoms reluctantly and seems embarrassed when Dr X asks him for details.

DESCRIBE

Problem

Mr D seems to have symptoms of panic disorder and OCD that interfere with his daily life and romantic relationships.

Patterns

*Mr D suffers from a lifelong pattern of low **self-esteem**. He feels unable to do things that other people can do, and he tends to withdraw from **relationships** when faced with **self-esteem threats**. Although he is interested in others and able to **empathize** with them, his relationships have lacked **security** and **intimacy**. Since grade school, he has had difficulty with **organizing** tasks and reading speed, although he has always excelled at math. He enjoys his **work** as a computer programmer but finds it difficult to relax on weekends and during vacations.*

REVIEW the developmental history

Mr D is the younger of two children whose parents are both highly educated professionals. His older sister always excelled at school and is now a physician. Mr D suffered from a learning disability and struggled academically despite receiving educational support and tutoring. Mr B felt that his parents, who highly valued academic achievement, always made him feel as though he were "defective" because of this, and felt that they favored his older, more successful sister.

Although Mr D first developed symptoms of anxiety in his early teens, he did not disclose this to anyone until his late 20s. Now, in his first significant romantic relationship, he is contemplating moving in with his girlfriend and is terrified about revealing his symptoms to her. Furthermore, he believes that "only people who are really ill take psychiatric medication." He feels that if he is prescribed a medication, it will signify that there is truly something wrong with him, and it will be one more thing that he has to hide from others, including his girlfriend. Also, he has heard that some medications used to treat OCD can cause low libido and impotence, and he is unwilling to consider a medication that could do that.

LINK problems/patterns to history

Mr D's low self-esteem may be related to his experience of his parents' attitudes toward him and his academically more successful sister, as well as to the difficulty he encountered in school. He has kept his symptoms a secret as a way to manage the shame he feels about them. He views medication as further evidence that he has something wrong with him, and this may influence his willingness to adhere to pharmacologic treatment. Mr D worries about potential sexual side effects of medication; therefore, if such symptoms were to develop, he might view them as a further, perhaps intolerable, blow to self-esteem.

This formulation helps Dr X to realize that in discussing a treatment plan with Mr D, it will be important to keep in mind Mr D's sensitivity about matters of self-esteem and his tendency not to reveal potentially shameful information about himself.

Now consider this formulation for Ms E:

Presentation

Ms E is a 45-year-old mother of two whose husband died of cancer a year and a half ago. She comes for a consultation with Dr W, a psychopharmacologist, at the suggestion of a friend who has benefited from medication for depression. Ms E has felt "under a lot of pressure" since her husband's death, has had trouble sleeping and concentrating, and feels "down" and often short-tempered. This is causing friction with her children at home and with colleagues at work, and she has fallen behind on professional obligations. She attributes these symptoms to her difficult life situation – that is, raising and supporting two children on her own. She tells Dr W that she's not sure if anyone, or anything, can help her and that she should just "pull myself together and get over it." When asked her thoughts about medication, Ms E says that she "wouldn't want to take anything that I could get addicted to." After the psychiatrist discusses the likelihood that an antidepressant medicine could help her to feel and function better, Ms E says, "Well, let's say that I do feel better – then what? Would I have to stay on the medicine for the rest of my life in order to function? I wouldn't want that."

DESCRIBE

Problem

Ms E has symptoms of depression in the context of a major loss, the death of her husband. She is ambivalent about considering medication treatment.

Patterns

*Ms E has generally had good **self-esteem** and has a **stable sense of identity**. Throughout her life she has had close friendships, characterized by **empathy** and **intimacy**, although she tends to prefer to rely on herself rather than on others. She feels that, before her husband's illness, she had a **mutually** satisfying relationship with him. She likes her **work** and believes that she does well at it, and, in the past, has enjoyed getting together with friends and reading.*

REVIEW the developmental history

Ms E grew up in a chaotic family, the oldest of four children. Her mother was addicted to alcohol and prescription drugs, and by the time Ms E was an early adolescent, her mother spent most of the time in her own bedroom. Her father was often away on business and was emotionally distant when home. Through most of her teenage years, Ms E was responsible for caring for her younger siblings and helping to run the household. Despite all of this, Ms E excelled at school and won a scholarship to a good college. After graduating she embarked on a successful career. She married in her mid-30s and had two children within a few years. She describes her late husband as a kind, loving, and trustworthy man, but says, "In the end, I couldn't depend on him, he got cancer and died."

LINK problems/patterns to history

Although Ms E appears to have considerable strengths, such as motivation, self-reliance, and resilience, which have helped her to establish a secure and successful life as an adult, she has had lifelong difficulty depending on others. Her early life history is notable for the lack of parental support, both emotional and practical, and her assumption of adult caregiving responsibilities while still in her teens. It is likely that her childhood experience of her parents as unreliable and undependable affected her attitude toward depending on others, a situation she mistrusts and avoids if possible. This attitude will likely influence her stance toward psychotropic medication and the doctor who prescribes it. Even if she agrees to try medication, and particularly if it helps her symptoms of depression, Ms E may remain highly ambivalent about remaining on medication.

Being able to formulate a theory about how her current attitudes about dependency developed over her lifetime, and how they influence her decision making about medication, may help Ms E to disentangle present-day choices from long-standing patterns of emotion and behavior.

21 Psychodynamic Formulation in Long-Term Psychodynamic Psychotherapy: Revising Over Time

Key concepts

When we conduct evaluations of patients, we construct initial psychodynamic formulations that help us to make treatment recommendations and guide our therapeutic strategy in the therapy.

In long-term psychodynamic psychotherapy, we continuously revise the formulation as we learn more about patients from

- how they see themselves in their outside lives
- new information that emerges in their life histories
- how they react to us in the context of the treatment

Formulations change over time

One of the most exciting and gratifying aspects of long-term psychodynamic psychotherapy is that it enables us to get to know patients very well over time. Week after week, we learn about our patients through what they say and how they behave. We learn about how they react to good news and bad news, excitement and stress, victories and losses. We learn about how they think and how they feel, how they love and how they hate. As our alliance with them grows, they tell us more about their lives, and, as they interact with us, we hypothesize about how they developed their unconscious fantasies and conflicts, relationship templates, sense of self, and attachment styles. We use this information to revise our initial formulation over time as we understand our patients, and their unconscious thoughts and feelings, more fully.

In this chapter, we will focus in detail on one psychodynamic psychotherapy in order to understand how a therapist's understanding of a person evolves during long-term treatment.

Psychodynamic Formulation, First Edition. Deborah L. Cabaniss, Sabrina Cherry, Carolyn J. Douglas, Ruth L. Graver, and Anna R. Schwartz.
© 2013 John Wiley & Sons, Ltd. Published 2013 by John Wiley & Sons, Ltd.

Initial presentation

Ms A, a 34-year-old divorced mother of a 4-year-old son, comes to see Mr Z seeking therapy to help her with stress related to managing her divorce and starting a new relationship. Ms A is an expressive, warm, and personable woman who says, "I really hope you can help me. I'm finally ready to try once and for all to figure this stuff out." She tells Mr Z that she and her now ex-husband, B, separated 2 years ago after she found out he was having an affair with a colleague. Ms A says that her husband was prone to angry outbursts and she thinks that it was the right decision to leave him. But she also says that the co-parenting has been difficult; her ex-husband travels a lot for work and, although he wants to co-parent, he often cancels visits with their son at the last minute. Ms A says her son is the "one good thing that came out of the marriage" and that he seems to be holding up well.

Ms A currently works as a software programmer. She has recently been promoted to a position in which she supervises a team of about 10 people. She enjoys her work and says, "Thank goodness for my job. I think it keeps me sane."

Ms A has begun a new relationship with C, a man who works at her company. While he is still married, C is separated from his wife and has hired a divorce lawyer. Ms A says that, in many ways, her relationship with C is an improvement over her relationship with her ex-husband. She thinks that C is kinder and more thoughtful than B, and she says that he can talk about his feelings and that he is less likely to fly off the handle. Ms A says she wants to stay in this relationship, but she is increasingly anxious about C's friendship with an ex-girlfriend who is now their colleague. She says she becomes intensely jealous whenever he mentions this colleague and remarks, "I'm afraid I'm going to sabotage this relationship."

When Mr Z asks her about her past psychiatric history, she says that she had several years of binging and purging in her early 20s that "went away on its own after I met my husband."

After Mr Z's first interview with Ms A, he conceptualizes her presenting **problems and patterns** in the following way:

DESCRIBE

Problem

Ms A is adjusting to being divorced. She wonders why she chose to marry a man who turned out to be so difficult. In addition, she has become increasingly jealous in her relationship with a new boyfriend.

Patterns

Self

*Ms A has a relatively positive **sense of her capabilities**, particularly at work. In the context of her relationships, however, Ms A is less secure and **more vulnerable to self-esteem threats**.*

Relationships

*Relationships are clearly the area in which Ms A has the most difficulty. Throughout her life, she has chosen to have relationships with people she is not fully able to **trust**, thus limiting the degree of **intimacy**, **security**, **and mutuality** she is able to experience. In her marriage, she chose to be with someone she now describes as angry and difficult. She is currently with a man who is not yet divorced and whose friendship with another woman makes her jealous. Her difficulty with relationships also seems to predate her marriage, since she is estranged from her older sister.*

Adapting

*Ms A tends to react quickly and somewhat **impulsively**. She is an **emotional** person who expresses her anger easily. At vulnerable times in her life (going to college, being on her own as a young adult), she has turned to action-oriented ways of handling her feelings (binging and purging). Of note, Ms A is able to handle her emotions far more effectively at work than in her personal relationships.*

Cognition

*Ms A's **cognitive functioning** is an area of strength. She performed well in school and has continued to advance at work. In addition, she has a good capacity for **self-reflection**. For example, she realizes that her jealousy about C is not fully rational and observes that she could be sabotaging the relationship.*

Work/play

*Ms A has found a **satisfying** career in which she is doing well. She enjoys being a parent and is relatively comfortable with her work/personal life balance.*

Based on this, Mr Z asks himself this focus question after his first interview with Ms A:

Why does Ms A repeatedly seem to choose relationships with men that do not provide the kind of intimacy she desires?

He hypothesizes that there are likely developmental explanations for this pattern, and as he reviews Ms A's history in his second evaluation session, he keeps this question in mind.

REVIEW the developmental history

Ms A says that she met normal developmental milestones and performed well in school. Her earliest memories are that her mother was warm and attentive. She describes her father as controlling and prone to angry outbursts, especially when he was drinking. He was occasionally physically abusive to her mother. Ms A says she "shut down" during these times and that her mother "tried her best to protect me but would ultimately give in to my father."

Ms A's parents have remained married. She says that her father has likely had affairs. Ms A is the middle of three sisters, each separated by 4 years. She reports that as children, the girls were close. Ms A feels that she was "always my father's favorite ... that drove my older sister crazy. I was better in school than she was and that went a long way with my father." As adults, the oldest sister and Ms A have had a falling-out. Ms A says "my sister never approved of my relationship with B so I couldn't bear talking to her."

Ms A says she has several close male friends but finds that for some reason her friendships with women "don't tend to last." Ms A had two serious relationships prior to meeting her husband; she says, "They were a lot like him – actually, they were probably worse. I seem to like intense, strong-minded men who aren't so good for me in the long run."

LINK

After their first two evaluation sessions, Mr Z organizes his mental notes and questions about the most important aspects of Ms A's psychology. Here's how he thinks about this as he writes his initial formulation:

*When I **describe Ms A's problems and patterns**, the area that stands out is relationships – that's where she's having the most difficulty. She repeatedly gets involved with people about whom she becomes jealous. Although she seems to be moving in the right direction – the relationship with C is better than the relationship with her husband – this pattern has repeated. She has many strengths – she has a good work history, enjoys being a parent, and is self-reflective.*

*What about her **history**? She seems to have had a secure attachment to her mother, but it sounds like things got more complicated in **middle childhood**. Being her father's favorite in the context of the parents' contentious relationship could not have been easy. That sounds like a trouble spot. Perhaps she had difficulties with triadic relationships; I think that I could **link** her relationship problems to her trouble in middle childhood using ideas about **conflict and defense** as an organizing idea. Her difficulties during this period may have led to her problems in romantic relationships later in life.*

Mr Z uses these points to develop his thinking about Ms A and writes the following formulation:

Initial psychodynamic formulation

Ms A has a strong positive sense of herself as evidenced by her confidence and enjoyment in her work and parenting. Her vulnerability to self-esteem threats is predominantly in relationship to other people. For example, Ms A could not tolerate her sister's criticism and therefore cut off contact with her.

Most significantly, Ms A's greatest difficulties are in the area of her intimate relationships. She realizes that when she married her husband, she chose a man remarkably like her father, and she wonders why she did that. The trouble that Ms A has in relationships often involves three people (herself, her partner, and a rival). This suggests that Ms A's difficulties with men could be related to problems with the three-person relationships of middle childhood. Ms A was her father's favorite – but she was the favorite of a man who was abusive to her mother. She may seek men like her father because she unconsciously continues to crave the admiration she felt for him. In addition, guilty feelings about devaluing her mother may have made her avoid competitive relationships with women, such as her relationship with her sister and with other female friends.

Use of the formulation

In the beginning of treatment

Mr Z's initial formulation suggests that Ms A has difficulty with three-person relationships and competitive anxiety because of unresolved unconscious conflicts. Mr Z decides to recommend twice-a-week psychodynamic psychotherapy that will encourage further exploration of her unconscious conflicts, perhaps in the context of the transference. Mr Z says to Ms A:

> *Your divorce has been a major event in your life and I can see that it is making you rethink a lot of things. I appreciate that you are noticing patterns in your relationships. I think you are asking a very important question when you wonder why you tend to get involved with difficult, angry men. This is something that we can try to figure out together in psychotherapy. You're aware of a lot about yourself – this will be helpful in this process. However, I think that you have thoughts and feelings that are out of awareness and are driving some of your choices. In therapy, we'll try to get as much access as we can to how your mind works and what you feel on a deeper level so that we can learn about what affects your decisions and choices. We can learn about your internal world from your thoughts and feelings about yourself, about people in your life, and even about me.*

Ms A begins twice-weekly psychotherapy, is able to talk in sessions, and is enthusiastic about treatment. As she engages in therapy, she talks less about her ex-husband and more about her relationship with C. In particular, she frequently mentions C's ex-girlfriend with whom she fears C will get back together – despite the fact that C has reassured her that there is no longer anything between them. Ms A confesses that she has begun to check C's computer for evidence of communication with his ex-girlfriend but so far has found nothing.

After a few months of treatment

Months go by and Mr Z begins wondering how Ms A's jealous and competitive feelings might emerge in her transference to him. He has been listening for hints about whether Ms A has been curious about who else he has in his life because three-person relationships appear to be central to her difficulties. About 6 months after starting therapy, right before Mr Z is going away for a 2-week vacation, Ms A has the following dream:

> Ms A   *It was winter and there was snow all around. I knocked on the door of a beautiful house.*
> *YOU answered the door! I said, "Hi, I'm here for the party." And you said, "Sorry, I*
> *think you got the date wrong." Then I heard your wife calling in the background,*
> *"Who is it honey?" And I felt so bad and started sobbing. That was the end of the dream.*

Mr Z thinks about the meaning of his upcoming vacation and wonders if perhaps Ms A is imagining with whom he will be when he is away. He says:

| Therapist | I wonder if my going away has something to do with this dream. Was there something about hearing my wife's voice in the dream that was upsetting to you? |
| Ms A | No, it wasn't that. It was that I had gotten the day wrong. I was so disappointed. I felt like I was being turned away into the cold. |

Mr Z's first response is to think that Ms A is not quite ready to talk about her feelings of jealousy toward important people in his life. He considers pursuing Ms A's feelings about the wife but notices that talking about "being turned away into the cold" has seemed to shake her up. Following the affect, he decides to ask about this:

Therapist	What about being turned away into the cold? Does that remind you of anything in particular?
Ms A	I felt so very sad. That house – it reminded me of the one I lived in when I was little, before my father started having trouble at work and we had to move to a smaller house. I remember there was this one winter, I was probably about 5 years old. There was more snow than usual and it was so cold, we couldn't go out. There was nothing to do. I was so lonely.
Therapist	Lonely?
Ms A	I don't know if I ever told you, but my mother got very depressed after my younger sister was born. The thing is, her mother, the grandmother I never met, died a few months before my sister was born. No one ever talks about it now but I think my mother might even have had to go to a hospital (Ms A starts to cry).
Therapist	Wow, it sounds like that was a very difficult time for you and your family.
Ms A	Yes, actually, now I'm thinking about it I don't know if my mother was ever really the same after that.

Mr Z mulls over this addition to Ms A's life story. He thinks more about what she has been discussing in recent weeks. He realizes that while initially focused on her jealousy about C's relationship with his ex-girlfriend, Ms A is now more preoccupied with details like how long it takes C to respond to her text messages, how many times they see each other in a week, and whether he remembers details about her life. Mr Z finds himself shifting his formulation toward considering Ms A's experience of her two-person relationships. In the next session, the last before Mr Z's vacation, Ms A starts by saying she's having a terrible time sleeping and that she is feeling very anxious. Mr Z decides to change his focus to see if this confirms his new viewpoint:

Therapist	I wonder if your trouble sleeping and your anxiety might be related to my going away for 2 weeks.
Ms A	Why are you going away anyway? What am I going to do without you? I feel like I might totally fall apart. It seems like we are just getting started. Why do you have to go away right now? Aren't therapists supposed to be there for their patients? I thought you really cared, but now I'm just not sure.
Therapist	You know, I wonder if this could have something to do with what we were talking about last time, about your mother's depression and when you felt so lonely without her. That must have been very scary.

Ms A   *Huh ... Maybe. I've been thinking a lot about it since our last meeting. I can't remember my mother being around much at all during those years. You know, my son is almost the same age I was back then. He needs me so much right now. How did I cope? I'm always there for him. And I don't just up and go on vacation.*

Ms A's response confirms Mr Z's evolving thoughts about Ms A. He thinks:

Ms A's reactions to me and the degree of anxiety she feels about my upcoming absence now seem less about jealousy or competitiveness and more about being taken care of by me. It's interesting the way that this vacation brought out that early memory about her mother. Both her reaction to me and this new information seem to confirm my thought that I had focused too much on Ms A's three-person relationships and not enough on her early dyadic relationship with her mother. I think that her earliest relationships weren't as secure as I thought they were. I think I'll revise the formulation, now using organizing ideas about attachment to link the problems/patterns to the history. Middle childhood relationships are also likely to have been problematic, but at this point in the treatment, it seems that thinking about attachment will help me more in trying to understand Ms A.

He revises his formulation as in the following.

Revised formulation from later in treatment

Ms A has a strong positive sense of herself as evidenced by her confidence and enjoyment in her work and as a parent. Her vulnerability to self-esteem threats is predominantly in relationship to other people. For example, Ms A could not tolerate her sister's criticism and therefore cut off contact with her. Ms A's greatest difficulties are in the area of her intimate relationships. It is likely that this is linked to difficulties that she had in her earliest relationships. Her mother, who was depressed from the time Ms A was aged 3 or 4 years, was unable to attend to her daughter's needs. There may even have been a period of separation. This led Ms A to develop an anxious attachment. This attachment style was compounded by her father's volatility and mother's submissive distress. In this context, she had difficulty developing certain central functions, including an ability to self-regulate and to modulate affect. As an adult, her preoccupied/anxious attachment style may make her unable to tolerate any absence from her partners, leading to continuous fears of abandonment. In addition, her difficulty with self-regulation may have led to her binging and purging behavior, as well as to her tendency to act impulsively. Ms A's middle childhood relationships were undoubtedly affected by her attachment style as well – she may have clung more desperately to her volatile but doting father, given her mother's emotional unavailability. This may have made it more difficult to identify with her mother and may have affected her ability to connect to women as an adult.

Using the revised formulation

Mr Z tells Ms A that he thinks this is an important phase in her therapy and that, although difficult, it will be helpful to her in understanding herself and her relationships. He reassures Ms A that there is a covering therapist whom she can call in his absence and that when he gets back, they will resume discussing these issues. Ms A seems calmer and wishes Mr Z a good vacation.

When Mr Z returns, he focuses on further understanding the period of Ms A's development during the time of her mother's depression. Ms A recounts that, around that time, she suffered stomachaches that caused her to miss many days of kindergarten, leaving her home with her mother who sat for long periods without talking. Ms A then talks more about her marriage and says, "You know, I think I sort of drove him crazy, always asking him when he'd be home. I used to get so mad if he was even 10 minutes later than he said he'd be." Mr Z helps Ms A to realize that she has a difficult time trusting her partner whenever he is away from her and that this is central to her relationship difficulties. As Ms A talks more about C, it becomes clear that her feelings about C's ex-girlfriend are less about jealousy and competition and more about wanting C's full attention. Mr Z is then able to help Ms A understand that this is a carryover from her feelings of longing for her mother. Over time, Ms A learns to trust that Mr Z cares about her and that he will reliably return from absences to resume their work together. This ultimately carries over to C, whom she also learns to trust and with whom she is able to have a closer, more mutually satisfying relationship.

In all of these situations, the formulation was central to the way the therapist planned and conducted the treatment. But how is the patient involved? When do we share our formulations? This is the subject of Chapter 22.

22 Sharing Formulations with Our Patients

Key concepts

Straightforward versions of our psychodynamic formulations can be helpful to patients in many instances including

- recommending treatment and setting early goals
- creating a life narrative
- offering explanation and perspective throughout the therapy
- consolidating insights as a preparation for termination

Timing is important when sharing a formulation.

It is important to anticipate our patients' reactions before we share the formulations with them and to monitor how they respond.

Formulations help us understand how our patients became who they are and how to focus the treatment. That's how they help US. But what about our patients? Do we share our formulations with them? Is it helpful to tell them how we think they became who they are or why they struggle with a given problem? When is it better to keep our formulations to ourselves? When working with patients, we constantly make choices about whether or not to share our hypotheses and, when we do, what to focus on. In this chapter, we review some principles for considering how and when to share our formulations with our patients.

How do we decide how and when to share formulations?

Learning about the way their development shaped their problems and patterns can help our patients to see themselves and their world in a new way. Thus, we need to share our formulations with them. But we need to think about how and when to do it. No patient needs to get a single-spaced typewritten formulation – rather, we share **parts** of our formulations, as they are relevant to what we are discussing in the treatment. We can use the same choosing principles that we use for deciding

---

Psychodynamic Formulation, First Edition. Deborah L. Cabaniss, Sabrina Cherry, Carolyn J. Douglas, Ruth L. Graver, and Anna R. Schwartz.

when and how to intervene to help us to think about how and when to share our formulations [28]. To review, these principles are

1. focus on material that is closest to the surface
2. follow the affect
3. listen to your countertransference

Are questions about his/her development on the surface of the patient's mind? Is the patient trying to make connections between his/her current life and the past? These could be good times to share parts of the formulation. On the other hand, moments of strong feelings about here-and-now situations, strong resistance to considering connections between the past and present, and points of weakened alliance are not likely to be opportune moments to share your formulation. Each situation is unique and the choosing principles are our guides.

Notice that we are talking about sharing "parts" of our formulations. Sharing our hypotheses about the developmental origins of a person's problems and patterns should help us to deepen the process, not to overwhelm or intellectualize it. Short segments of formulation that are directly related to what is uppermost in the patient's mind are most likely to have a therapeutic effect. Sharing formulations can "backfire" if we say too much, are not attuned to the current affect, or try to impose hypotheses on patients who are not open to new views about themselves. Patients with self-esteem problems and/or long-standing, difficult interpersonal relationship patterns may experience even the most gently worded formulations as critical. As therapists, we have to be aware of this possibility and to carefully monitor our patient's reactions to the pieces of formulation we share. Consider this example:

Ms A is an 80-year-old woman who presents for help with feelings of loneliness and depression. She has two sons who are married with established families of their own, living across the country. She explains that now that airplane travel is more difficult for her, she doesn't see them as much as she'd like. She feels alone and upset that her children live so far away. She worries that they do not love her. She no longer calls them because she feels she is intruding into their lives, which makes her feel even more alone and isolated. As she tells her history, she reports that she has suffered multiple abandonments in her life – her mother was depressed and hospitalized off and on throughout her youth, and her husband died from lung cancer in his 40s, leaving her to raise her sons alone. She never married again because she did not want to risk having another ill husband. She was independent, kept to herself, asked little of her children as they grew up, and acted as if family ties were unimportant. She believed that one's children should "live their own lives."

The therapist formulates that Ms A has an avoidant attachment style, stemming from her own experience with a depressed, emotionally unavailable mother. The therapist notes that Ms A has tried to live without relying on others and acts as if she expects little from her family. Now, in her 80s, she feels abandoned and hurt but acts as if she is not interested in making contact. The therapist shares this formulation with Ms A, saying, "Ever since your husband died you have acted as if you are fine on your own and expect little from your children. While they have grown up nicely, this approach has given them the signal that you do not need very much from them. This is a strategy you developed in childhood as an approach to your mother's depression and the independence you had to achieve as a child, and that you used again after your husband passed away, but it is no longer working for you, since you actually would like more connection with your children and their families at this juncture."

> *The formulation, although likely accurate, makes Ms A feel as if it is her fault that she has no connection to her children and she states, "You're right, I have really messed this all up and they do not like me or wish to be with me. I have raised selfish children. I guess I deserve to die alone."*

In this case, the patient experienced the therapist's formulation as further evidence of her own bad feelings about herself. While this was not the therapist's intention, hearing the patient's reaction to the formulation helped her to experience firsthand the way the patient contributes to her negative self-perception. Even when we carefully consider how and when to share our formulations, we will not always get it right, but if we listen to our patients' reactions, it will always help us to deepen the treatment.

Situations in which sharing formulations is particularly helpful

There are several treatment situations in which sharing formulations is particularly helpful:

Making treatment recommendations

An internist tells a cancer patient his diagnosis and then makes a recommendation for surgery or chemotherapy, citing the available evidence. If the patient asks why he has cancer, the doctor shares current knowledge about risk factors and etiology. When recommending psychotherapy, it is also important to tell the patient how we understand the problem, what treatments are available, and why we chose the treatment. This can involve sharing part of the initial psychodynamic formulation to help patients understand that unconscious factors may play a role in their difficulties. Here is an example:

> *Ever since bringing his youngest daughter to college 2 weeks ago, Mr B has been unable to sleep. He states that he was looking forward to the "empty nest" to take a trip with his wife and to do more socializing with friends, but that he is too exhausted to do much of anything. When he tells his history, he reports that his parents were in an unhappy marriage and waited to separate until after he went to college. He feels lucky that he loves his wife.*

Toward the end of the session, the therapist, who is also a psychiatrist, offers Mr B some advice about sleep hygiene and gives him a prescription for a sleeping pill, offering the appropriate instruction on its safe use. In addition, the therapist says:

> *While the pills will likely enable you to sleep, it sounds like you have some real feelings about your daughter leaving home, even though you have been looking forward to this time with your wife. It is possible that the feelings you have about your own parents' divorce are affecting your ability to transition into this next phase of your life. I think that talking about this in psychotherapy will help you to understand this additional part of what you are going through. This course of psychotherapy should not only help with your current symptoms but also give you some insights that will help you to enjoy what you have ahead.*

In this example, the therapist hypothesizes that taking his daughter to college has caused Mr B to activate unconscious feelings that he is having about his parents' divorce and that this is affecting his ability to sleep. The therapist describes the problem (difficulty with loss and moving forward), reviews the history (parental divorce at a similar time of life), and uses ideas about the impact of early relationships, conflicts, and defenses to link history to development (defense against experiencing the loss of his daughter because it reminds him of a painful loss from the past). The therapist keeps this more technical version of the formulation in his mind, while translating it into straightforward language that the patient can understand. This allows Mr B to get a better sense of his current situation, as well as a clear idea of why the therapist is recommending psychotherapy.

Generating a life narrative

For many patients, being able to construct a narrative of how they came to be the way they are can be very therapeutic. It can often help them to gain perspective, particularly at difficult moments of their lives. Sharing our formulations with our patients can help them to create and revise their life narratives [12]. Continuing with Mr B:

> As the psychotherapy sessions continue, it becomes clear that, after his parent's divorce, Mr B's mother was very unhappy and took a long time to make a new life for herself. In college, Mr B remained dedicated to his mother, making frequent trips home to keep her company. He recapitulates this pattern in his current life, often denying his own difficulties in order to be strong for others. For example, he has supported his depressed wife for years, and he is the parent who helps his daughter when she is overwhelmed by schoolwork. This further history suggests that Mr B may be having difficulty dealing with his feelings about his daughter's transition because he continues to feel that he needs to be positive and to support others.

The therapist now has an understanding of Mr B's defenses against the experience of loss that goes beyond the initial formulation. He thinks that sharing this aspect of the formulation with Mr B may help him to understand his trouble with grieving. The therapist says:

> One reason why you may be having trouble moving into the next phase of your life is that you are actually very sad that your daughter has left home. You are usually the one called on to "look at the bright side" – whether that was to help your mother after the divorce or to help build your wife's and daughter's confidence. You are the upbeat one, so you naturally want to think about what fun you can have traveling with your wife, rather than pause to allow yourself to be sad that your daughter has left. All of your life you have helped others manage their pain, but now you are in pain and you don't know how to depend on someone emotionally to work this through. In some ways, this therapy is a first step at learning how to do this.

In response, Mr B says

> You're right, that's the story of my life. I learned to be that way in my relationship with my mother, and I've repeated it in my relationship with my wife and my daughter. It's a nice way to be, and I'm sure that I'll always help them in that way, but I think that it has made it difficult for me to be sad now.

By sharing his formulation, the therapist is helping Mr B to generate his life narrative. This will help Mr B to understand his past, his present, and his future.

Fostering insight during the treatment

By offering a developmental perspective, sharing our formulations can also help patients who face difficult insights about themselves in therapy. For example:

> During a therapy session, a patient feels acutely guilty as she realizes that she has been overly harsh with her daughter. The therapist says, "I know that you feel very bad about your behavior, but it sounds like you learned from your mother to have very high standards and that you were never allowed any flexibility. That was the only model you knew."

This simple formulation, which traces a current problem to an early relationship template, links the patient's current behavior toward her daughter to her mother's behavior toward her. It helps the patient not only to understand the etiology of her behavior but also to recognize why she is so hard on herself. These insights can help to alleviate the patient's guilt, making her more able to work on these issues in treatment and helping her to improve her relationship with her daughter.

Preparing the patient for termination

Termination is another time when sharing formulations can be helpful in the treatment process. During the end phase of therapy, it is often helpful to give patients explanatory summaries that they can take with them, reminding them of what they have learned about themselves. Often, these summary statements help patients to mark the work they have done in therapy and to feel more confident about confronting new situations in the future. Consider Mr B, whose daughter just left for college and who learned in therapy that he is more comfortable helping others than taking care of himself. After benefitting enormously from the treatment, Mr B is ready to terminate the therapy. In one of the final sessions, his therapist decides to share some of the formulation with him, saying

> As we've learned, your most comfortable stance with other people has been to be the strong one. You developed this approach to manage your own sadness in childhood when your parents were unhappy with each other, and again later when they divorced. You continued this strategy to help your mother after your father left, to help your wife with her depression, and to support your daughter with her academic challenges. While this "worked" for many years, it left you without the ability to lean on others when you were in need. When you came to see me you were sad but didn't know it – you experienced it as an inability to sleep. Our therapy was the first time you really sought help for a problem of your own, and your ability to allow yourself to work with me has really helped you. In recent months, you've been much more able to communicate your needs to your wife, and even to some friends. Going forward, this will help you enormously. It's possible that in the future, you may have another situation in which you have some kind of symptom – it could be insomnia again, or something else. If this happens, you are welcome to return to therapy, but you might also consider what we've learned together and ask yourself whether you are in need of support from the people around you.

This piece of formulation helps Mr B to consolidate what he has learned and to think about possible problem spots that could arise in the future. In this way, our psychodynamic formulations will stay with our patients, reminding them of their work with us and helping them with new situations and transitions for the rest of their lives.

Part Five References

1. Gorton GE. Commentary: Psychodynamic approaches to the patient. *Psychiatric Services* 2000; **51**: 1408–1409.
2. Talbott JA. Crisis intervention and psychoanalysis: Compatible or antagonistic? *Psychoanalytic Psychotherapy* 1980; **8**: 189–201.
3. Myerson AT, Glick RA. The use of psychoanalytic concepts in crisis intervention. *Psychoanalytic Psychotherapy* 1980; **8**: 171–188.
4. Blackman JS. Psychodynamic techniques during urgent consultation interviews. *The Journal of Psychotherapy Practice and Research* 1994; **3**: 194–203.
5. MacKinnon RA, Michels R, Buckley PJ. The emergency patient. In: *The Psychiatric Interview in Clinical Practice*. American Psychiatric Publishing, Inc.: Washington, DC, 2006: 481–504.
6. Silbert H. The emergency room. In: Schwartz HJ, Bleiberg E, Weissman SH (eds.). *Psychodynamic Concepts in General Psychiatry*. American Psychiatric Publishing, Inc.: Washington, DC, 1995: 49–68.
7. Sulkowicz K. Psychodynamic issues in the emergency department. *Psychiatric Clinics of North America* 1999; **22**: 911–922.
8. Leibenluft E, Tasman A, Green SA. *Less Time to Do More: Psychotherapy on the Short-Term Inpatient Unit*. American Psychiatric Publishing, Inc.: Washington, DC, 1993.
9. Wolpert EA. The inpatient unit. In: Schwartz HJ, Bleiberg E, Weissman SH (eds.). *Psychodynamic Concepts in General Psychiatry*. American Psychiatric Publishing, Inc.: Washington, DC, 1995: 39–48.
10. Gabbard GO. *Psychodynamic Psychiatry in Clinical Practice*. American Psychiatric Publishing, Inc.: Washington, DC, 1995.
11. Viederman M. The psychodynamic consultation. In: Barnhill JW (ed). *Approach to the Psychiatric Patient: Case-Based Essays*. American Psychiatric Publishing, Inc.: Washington, DC, 2009: 183–185.
12. Viederman M. The psychodynamic life narrative: A psychotherapeutic intervention useful in crisis situations. *Psychiatry* 1983; **46**: 236–246.
13. Blumenfeld M. The place of psychodynamic psychiatry in consultation-liaison psychiatry with special emphasis on countertransference. *Journal of the American Academy of Psychoanalysis and Dynamic Psychiatry* 2006; **34**: 83–92.
14. Lefer J. The psychoanalyst at the medical bedside. *Journal of the American Academy of Psychoanalysis and Dynamic Psychiatry* 2006; **34**: 75–81.
15. Barnhill JW. Overview of hospital psychodynamics. In: Barnhill J (ed). *Approach to the Psychiatric Patient: Case-Based Essays*. American Psychiatric Publishing, Inc.: Washington, DC, 2009: 207–210.
16. Strain JJ, Grossman S. *Psychological Care of the Medically Ill: A Primer in Liaison Psychiatry*. Appleton-Century-Crofts and Fleschner: New York, 1975.
17. Muskin PR. The combined use of psychotherapy and pharmacology in the medical setting. *Psychiatric Clinics of North America* 1990; **13**: 341–353.
18. MacKinnon RA, Michels R, Buckley PJ. The hospitalized patient. In: *The Psychiatric Interview in Clinical Practice*. American Psychiatric Publishing, Inc.: Washington, DC, 2006: 505–520.
19. Muskin PR. The medical hospital. In: Schwartz HJ, Bleiberg E, Weissman SH (eds.). *Psychodynamic Concepts in General Psychiatry*, 4th edn. American Psychiatric Publishing, Inc.: Washington, DC, 1995: 69–88.
20. Grossman S. The use of psychoanalytic theory and technique on the medical ward. *Psychoanalytic Psychotherapy* 1984; **10**: 533–548.
21. Nash SS, Kent LK, Muskin PR. Psychodynamics in medically ill patients. *Harvard Review of Psychiatry* 2009; **17** (6): 389–397.

22. Schwartz HJ. Introduction. In: Schwartz HJ, Bleiberg E, Weissman SH (eds.). *Psychodynamic Concepts in General Psychiatry*. American Psychiatric Publishing, Inc.: Washington, DC, 1995: xix–xxi.

23. Shapiro ER. Management vs. interpretation: Teaching residents to listen. *The Journal of Nervous and Mental Disease* 2012; **200** (3): 204–207.

24. Mojtabai R, Olfson M. National trends in psychotherapy by office-based psychiatrists. *Archives of General Psychiatry* 2008; **65** (8): 962–970.

25. Gabbard GO. Deconstructing the "med check." *Psychiatric Times* 2009; **26** (9) *www .psychiatrictimes.com/display/article/10168/1444238*.

26. Plakun E. Treatment resistance and psychodynamic psychiatry: Concepts psychiatry needs from psychoanalysis. *Psychodynamic Psychiatry* 2012; **40** (2): 183–210.

27. Mintz D, Belnap BA. What is psychodynamic psychopharmacology? An approach to pharmacologic treatment resistance. In: Plakun E (ed). *Treatment Resistance and Patient Authority: The Austen Riggs Reader*. W.W. Norton & Co.: New York, 2011.

28. Cabaniss DL, Cherry S, Douglas CJ *et al*. *Psychodynamic Psychotherapy: A Clinical Manual*. Wiley-Blackwell: Oxford, 2011.

29. Zeber J, Copeland LA, Good CB *et al*. Therapeutic alliance perceptions and medication adherence in patients with bipolar disorder. *Journal of Affective Disorders* 2008; **107**: 53–62.

30. Skodol AE, Grilo CM, Keyes K *et al*. Relationship of personality disorders to the course of major depressive disorder in a nationally representative sample. *American Journal of Psychiatry* 2011; **168**: 257–264.

31. Skodol AE, Gunderson JG, Shea MT *et al*. The collaborative longitudinal personality disorders study (CLPS): Overview and implications. *Journal of Personality Disorders* 2005; **19**: 487–504.

32. Busch, FN, Auchincloss EL. The psychology of prescribing and taking medication. In: Schwartz H, Bleiberg E, Weissman S (eds.). *Psychodynamic Concepts in General Psychiatry*. American Psychiatric Publishing, Inc.: Arlington, 1995: 401–416.

33. Busch FN, Sandberg LS. *Psychotherapy and Medication: The Challenge of Integration*. Analytic Press: New York, 2007.

34. Frank AF, Gunderson JG. The role of the therapeutic alliance in the treatment of schizophrenia: Relationship to course and outcome. *Archives of General Psychiatry* 1990; **47** (3): 228–236.

35. Douglas CJ. Teaching supportive psychotherapy to psychiatric residents. *American Journal of Psychiatry* 2008; **165**: 445–452.

Epilogue

A new set of clinical skills

By reading this book, you have learned a new set of valuable clinical skills. You've learned how to describe a person's problems and patterns, to take a comprehensive history, and to link them using organizing ideas about development to construct a psychodynamic formulation. We hope that we've demonstrated that you can use these skills with all of your patients in any treatment setting – short term and long term, inpatient and outpatient, and solo and combined with medication.

If you're a trainee, you may be asked to write psychodynamic formulations for your classes, for supervision, or for case conferences. Doing this will help you to hone your skills. Sharing formulations with your peers can be extremely useful, allowing you to learn from their experiences and ideas. Sharing formulations with supervisors generally enriches the supervisory experience. If it's a short-term supervision, writing an initial formulation can help you to discuss treatment goals and therapeutic strategy. If it's a long-term supervision, writing annual formulations can help you to evolve and shape your ideas about the treatment as you get to know the patient better and gain new understanding of him/her.

If you're no longer a trainee, having the discipline to actually write formulations may be harder. As we mentioned in Chapter 1, we suggest that you try to write a few formulations in order to practice your skills. Even if you think that you have an idea of your formulation, putting pen to paper forces you to really examine what you think and how you understand your patients and their development. Once you've done that, you can decide how writing formulations will fit into your practice. You may want to write psychodynamic formulations for all of your patients, or you may want to jot down ideas about the formulation as they come up and change. Often, writing a formulation can help you to figure out a difficult moment in a treatment, understand your countertransference, or prepare for a consultation with a colleague or supervisor. Regardless of the way you decide to use formulations in your practice, you have gained an important skill that can enhance all of your clinical work.

Psychodynamic Formulation, First Edition. Deborah L. Cabaniss, Sabrina Cherry, Carolyn J. Douglas, Ruth L. Graver, and Anna R. Schwartz.
© 2013 John Wiley & Sons, Ltd. Published 2013 by John Wiley & Sons, Ltd.

A new way to understand your patients

Of course, the primary reason we formulate psychodynamically is to help our patients. When we know what their difficulties are and how they developed, we are in the best position to recommend and carry out treatments that can help them to develop new and more adaptive ways of thinking about themselves, relating to others, and adapting to stress. Ultimately, psychodynamic psychotherapy is about new growth and development. Only by knowing how and why our patients' developmental paths stalled or went awry can we work with them to create new ways of thinking about themselves and others and adapting to their world.

From formulation to treatment

In this book, we've linked patterns with history; now we can link formulation to treatment. Although we have briefly addressed the ways in which formulating guides the way we plan and conduct treatment, we suggest that you now learn more about psychodynamic techniques in *Psychodynamic Psychotherapy: A Clinical Manual*. The patterns that we've described here all correspond to the major treatment strategies that we have outlined in the *Manual*.

An invitation to curiosity

As we've said, there are no formulations without questions. Only by continuing to ask questions about our patients – about why they think, feel, and behave the way they do – can we help them with the things that make them suffer. So be curious. Wonder. Contemplate. Hypothesize. Revise. We hope that the skills that you have learned in this book – describing, reviewing, and linking – will help you to keep trying to answer these questions in your work with patients. Endless questions, endless formulations – endlessly interesting!

Appendix – How to Use *Psychodynamic Formulation*: A Guide for Educators

As we mentioned in the Introduction, we do not teach psychodynamic formulation all at once. Our aim is to help students feel that constructing psychodynamic formulations is an automatic and natural part of treating patients, rather than an onerous task that they will only do once in their lives. Thus, we teach this process in a gradual way that allows them to consolidate learning without feeling overwhelmed.

Learning to construct psychodynamic formulations is a multistep process. It requires students to learn how to

- DESCRIBE problems and patterns (including asking questions about general functioning)
- REVIEW developmental histories (including taking a developmental history from an adult patient)
- LINK problems and patterns to history (including focusing on what they have DESCRIBED and REVIEWED and choosing useful ideas about development)
- use psychodynamic formulations to guide treatment

Each of these steps requires different kinds of learning and is appropriate for different phases of training. The following are some suggestions about how to teach each of these steps in a mental health training program:

DESCRIBE

Whether or not your junior trainees are seeing patients in psychodynamic psychotherapy, if they are in a clinical training program they are seeing *patients*. This is a good time to begin to introduce them to DESCRIBING. Many of them are used to thinking

Psychodynamic Formulation, First Edition. Deborah L. Cabaniss, Sabrina Cherry, Carolyn J. Douglas, Ruth L. Graver, and Anna R. Schwartz.
© 2013 John Wiley & Sons, Ltd. Published 2013 by John Wiley & Sons, Ltd.

about making DSM diagnoses – having them begin to think beyond disorders is the first step toward getting them to think psychodynamically. You can begin by teaching the difference between the **Problem** and the **Person**. Next, try introducing the five patterns – SELF, RELATIONSHIPS, ADAPTING, COGNITION, and WORK AND PLAY. Chapters 4–8 are appropriate for this teaching. In a 4-year psychiatry residency, we teach this material in our PG-II year (suggested time frame: 4–8 weeks).

Suggested activities

1. **Problem/Person exercise** – Have students do a writing exercise in which they describe the **Problem** and the **Person** for one of their patients. This can be any patient whom they have seen recently (no more than one page).

2. **DESCRIBE "putting it together" exercise** – Have students describe the five patterns: SELF, RELATIONSHIPS, ADAPTING, COGNITION, and WORK/PLAY for one of their patients. Encourage them to write each section separately, trying to address each variable. Share work in class so that students are exposed to a range of patients.

3. **Interview patients in class** and have students generate DESCRIBE sections in small groups.

REVIEW

Junior trainees can also learn to REVIEW. This involves more than simply teaching development; students need to learn how to take developmental histories from adult patients. It also involves helping students correlate certain developmental periods with particular adult problems and patterns. Chapters 9–12 are appropriate for this teaching, which can be taught in the PG-II or early PG-III year (suggested time frame: 4–8 weeks).

Suggested activities

1. **REVIEW "putting it together" exercise** – Have students write a REVIEW section for one of their patients. As with DESCRIBE, try to have them use the headers so that they include all phases of development. Share work among students (no longer than three pages).

2. **DESCRIBE + REVIEW exercise** – Students can now begin to put two sections together for the same patient.

3. **Vignettes** – Write vignettes about common adult presentations and have students work in groups during class to think about when patients might have had difficulty during development.

Organizing ideas about development

Although mental health trainees are often champing at the bit to learn about "theory," learning this too early can lead to intellectualization in formulation and treatment.

Therefore, we wait until slightly later in training to introduce this (PG-III year). Again, learning in this area involves more than just becoming familiar with the different organizing ideas; it also requires guidance about how to choose the ones that will be most useful for explaining certain clinical situations. Chapters 13–18 are appropriate for this teaching (suggested time frame: 8 weeks).

Suggested activities

Choosing ideas about development

1. **Group work** – With vignettes or videos of psychotherapy sessions, use group discussion to consider how clinical situations might be understood using different ideas about development.

2. **Individual work** – Have students write up a short clinical situation using two different ideas about development.

LINK

Once students have learned to DESCRIBE and REVIEW, and have been introduced to the organizing ideas about development, it's time to teach LINKING. You can use the model outlined in the Introduction to Part Four for this teaching. The skills involved are learning to focus on what they have DESCRIBED and REVIEWED, asking a focus question, choosing organizing ideas for linking, and writing a chronological narrative. The examples in Chapters 13–18 can serve as guides, as can the "Putting It Together" example from Part Four. This teaching is best reserved for more senior trainees – we teach it in the second half of the PG-III year (suggested time frame: 4–8 weeks). This section can culminate in writing and sharing full formulations.

Suggested activities

1. **Focusing DESCRIBE and REVIEW** – Offer students sample DESCRIBE and REVIEW segments and have them identify the areas they think should be the focus.

2. **Forming questions** – Have students describe patient presentations and ask the group to suggest focus questions that they would like to answer with a psychodynamic formulation.

3. **"Putting it together"** – Have students write DESCRIBE, REVIEW, and LINK sections for one of their patients. Involve supervisors in this project. Have the students read each others' work. In class, students can discuss the choices they made about focusing and choosing ideas about development. This helps the groups to learn about different ways of LINKING and exposes them to more psychodynamic formulations.

Using formulations to guide treatment

Once students have written their own psychodynamic formulations, they can begin to think about how to use them to guide treatment. For this, it is important to enlist the help of the clinical supervisors. Chapters 2 and 19–22 are appropriate for this teaching. Areas to emphasize include goal setting and making treatment recommendations, using psychodynamic formulations in different clinical settings, termination, and revising formulations over time. This teaching can begin in the middle of training and continue forever.

Suggested activities

1. **Have a faculty development workshop** – Bring your clinical supervisors together to discuss writing and using psychodynamic formulations in training. Consider doing some of the above exercises with the supervisors so that they can have a sense of what and how the students are learning.

2. **Learn about formulating in other treatment modalities** – Have educators from other treatment areas (psychopharmacology and other psychotherapies) teach together so students can learn about different ways of formulating – often for the same patients.

Recommended Reading

Recommended Reading: Part One

Chapters 1–3

1. Cabaniss DL, Cherry S, Douglas CJ, Schwartz AR. *Psychodynamic Psychotherapy: A Clinical Manual*. Wiley-Blackwell: Oxford, 2011.
2. Campbell WH, Rohrbaugh, RM. *The Biopsychosocial Formulation Manual*. Routledge: New York, 2006.
3. Eels TD (ed). *Handbook of Psychotherapy Case Formulation*. Guilford Press: New York, 2007.
4. Friedman RS, Lister P. The current status of psychodynamic formulation. *Psychiatry* 1987; **50** (2): 126–141.
5. Kassaw K, Gabbard GO. Creating a pychodynamic formulation from a clinical evaluation. *American Journal of Psychiatry* 2002; **159**: 721–726.
6. MacKinnon RA, Yudofsky SC. *The Psychiatric Evaluation in Clinical Practice*. J.B. Lippincott Company: Philadelphia, 1986.
7. McWilliams N. *Psychoanalytic Case Formulation*. Guilford Press: New York, 1999.
8. Perry S, Cooper AM, Michels R. The psychodynamic formulation: Its purpose, structure, and clinical application. *The American Journal of Psychiatry* 1987; **144**: 543–550.
9. Summers RF, Barber JP. *Psychodynamic Therapy: A Guide to Evidence-Based Practice*. Guilford Press: New York, 2010.

Recommended Reading: Part Two

Chapter 4

1. Erikson E. *Identity: Youth and Crisis*. W.W. Norton & Co.: New York, 1968.
2. Kohut H, Wolff ES. The disorder of the self and their treatment, an outline. *International Journal of Psychoanalysis* 1978; **59**: 413–414.
3. Kernberg OF. Factors in the psychoanalytic treatment of narcissistic personalities. *Journal of the American Psychoanalytic Association* 1970; **18**: 51–85.
4. Sandler J, Holder A, Meers D. The ego ideal and the ideal self. *Psychoanalytic Study of the Child* 1963; **18**: 139–158.

Psychodynamic Formulation, First Edition. Deborah L. Cabaniss, Sabrina Cherry, Carolyn J. Douglas, Ruth L. Graver, and Anna R. Schwartz.
© 2013 John Wiley & Sons, Ltd. Published 2013 by John Wiley & Sons, Ltd.

Chapter 5

1. Beebe B, Lachman FM. The contribution of mother-infant mutual influence to the origins of self and object representation. *Psychoanalytic Psychology* 1988; **5**: 305–337.
2. Bowlby J. The nature of the child's tie to his mother. *International Journal of Psychoanalysis* 1958; **39**: 350–373.
3. Bowlby J. *Attachment, Vol. 1 of Attachment and Loss*. Basic Books: New York, 1982.
4. Greenberg JR, Mitchell SA. *Object Relations in Psychoanalytic Theory*. Harvard University Press: Cambridge, 1983.
5. Slade A. Attachment theory and research: Implications for the theory and practice of individual psychotherapy with adults. In: Cassidy J, Shaver PR (eds.). *Handbook of Attachment: Theory, Research and Clinical Applications*. Guilford Press: New York, 2008: 762–782.
6. Stern DN. *The Interpersonal World of the Infant*. Basic Books: New York, 1985.

Chapter 6

1. Freud S. The neuro-psychoses of defense. In: Strachey, J (ed). *The Standard Edition of the Complete Psychological Works of Sigmund Freud, Volume III (1893-1899), Early Psycho-Analytic Publications*. Hogarth Press: London, 1894: 41–61.
2. Gabbard GO. *Psychodynamic Psychiatry in Clinical Practice*, 4th edn. American Psychiatric Publishing, Inc.: Washington, DC, 2005.
3. Kernberg OF. *Object-Relations Theory and Clinical Psychoanalysis*. Aronson: New York, 1976.
4. Shapiro D. *Neurotic Styles*. Basic Books: New York, 1973.
5. Vaillant GE. *Adaptation to Life How the Best and the Brightest Came of Age*, 1st edn. Little, Brown & Co.: Boston, 1977.

Chapter 7

1. Allen JG. Mentalizing. In: Allen JG, Fonagy P (eds.). *Practice in Handbook of Mentalization-Based Treatment*. Wiley: Oxford, 2006: 3–30.
2. Clarkin JF, Howieson DB, McClough J. The role of psychiatric measures in assessment and treatment. In: Hales RE, Yudofsky SC, Gabbard GO (eds.). *American Psychiatric Publishing Textbook of Psychiatry*, 5th edn. American Psychiatric Publishing, Inc.: Washington, DC, 2008: 73–112.
3. Coltart NE. Assessment of psychological mindedness in the clinical interview. *British Journal of Psychiatry* 1988; **153**: 819–820.
4. Folstein MF, Folstein SE, McHugh PR. 'Mini-mental state'. A practical method for grading the cognitive state of patients for the physician. *Journal of Psychiatric Research* 1975; **12**: 189–198.
5. Fonagy P. Thinking about thinking: Some clinical and theoretical considerations in the treatment of a borderline patient. *International Journal of Psychoanalysis* 1991; **72**: 639–656.
6. Goldstein G. Cognitive assessment with adults. In: Thomas JC, Hersen M (eds.). *Handbook of Clinical Psychology Competencies*. Springer: New York, 2010: 237–260.
7. Hall JA. Psychological-mindedness: A conceptual model. *American Journal of Psychotherapy* 1992; **46** (1): 131–140.
8. Lichter, DG, Cummings JL. *Psychiatric and Neurological Disorders*. Guilford Press: New York, 2001.
9. Roberts AC, Robbins TW, Weiskrantz L. *The Prefrontal Cortex: Executive and Cognitive Functions*. Oxford University Press: Oxford, 2002.

10. Taylor GJ. Psychoanalysis and empirical research: The example of patients who lack psychological-mindedness. *Journal of the American Academy of Psychoanaylsis* 1995; **23**: 263–281.

Chapter 8

1. Brown S. *Play: How it Shapes the Brain, Opens the Imagination, and Invigorates the Soul*. Penguin Books: New York, 2009.
2. DeLamater J. Sexual expression in later life: A review and synthesis. *The Journal of Sex Research* 2012; **49** (2–3): 125–141.
3. Paluska SA, Schwenk TL. Physical activity and mental health. *Sports Medicine* 2000; **29** (3): 167–180.
4. Terr L. *Beyond Love and Work: Why Adults Need to Play*. Touchstone: New York, 1999.

Recommended Reading: Part Three

Chapter 9

1. Burmeister M, McInnis MG, Zöllner S. Psychiatric genetics: Progress amid controversy. *Nature Reviews Genetics* 2008; **9** (7): 527–540.
2. Dunkel Schetter C, Tanner, L. Anxiety, depression and stress in pregnancy: Implications for mothers, children, research, and practice, *Current Opinion in Psychiatry* 2012; **25** (2): 141–148.
3. Minnes S, Lang A, Singer L. Prenatal tobacco, marijuana, stimulant, and opiate exposure: Outcomes and practice implications. *Addiction Science & Clinical Practice* 2011; **6** (1): 57–70.
4. Riley EP, Infante A, Warren KR. Fetal alcohol spectrum disorders: An overview. *Neuropsychology Review* 2011; **21** (2): 73–80.

Chapter 10

1. Ainsworth MDS, Blehar MC, Waters E *et al*. *Patterns of Attachment: A Psychological Study of the Strange Situation*. Erlbaum: Hillsdale, NJ, 1978.
2. Bateman A, Fonagy P. Mentalizing and borderline personality disorder. In: Allen JG, Fonagy P (eds.). *Handbook of Mentalization Based Treatment* Wiley: Hoboken, NJ, 2006: 185–200.
3. Beebe B, Lachmann F. *Infant Research and Adult Treatment: Co-Constructing Interactions*. Analytic Press: Hillsdale, NJ, 2002.
4. Main M. Recent studies in attachment: Overview, with selected implications for clinical work. In: Goldberg S, Muir R, Kerr J (eds.). *Attachment Theory: Social, Developmental and Clinical Perspectives*. Analytic Press: Hillsdale, NJ, 1995: 407–474.
5. Winnicott DW. *The Maturational Processes and the Facilitating Environment* Hogarth Press: London, 1965.
6. Davies D. *Child Development: A Practitioner's Guide*. Guilford Press: New York, 2011.

Chapter 11

1. Freud S. Three essays on the theory of sexuality. In: Strachey, J (ed). *The Standard Edition of the Complete Psychological Works of Sigmund Freud, Volume VII (1901-1905): A Case of Hysteria, Three Essays on Sexuality and Other Works*. Hogarth Press: London, 1905: 123–246.

2. Isay R. *Being Homosexual: Gay Men and their Development*. Farrar Strauss Giroux: New York, 1989.
3. Roiphe H, Roiphe A. *Your Child's Mind*. St. Martin's Press: New York; 1985.
4. Sophocles. *The Three Theban Plays*. Penguin Books: New York, 1982.

Chapter 12

1. Beardslee WR, Valliant G. Adult development. In: Tasman A, Kay J, Lieberman JA *et al.* (eds.). *Psychiatry*, 3rd edn. Wiley: Oxford, 2008: 181–195.
2. Bienenfeld D. Late life. In: Tasman A, Kay J, Lieberman JA *et al.* (eds.). *Psychiatry*, 3rd edn. Wiley: London, 2008: 196–202.
3. Erikson E. *Childhood and Society*, 2nd edn. W.W. Norton & Co.: New York, 1963.
4. Pruitt D. *Your Adolescent*. HarperCollins: New York, 1999.
5. Shapiro T, Amso D. School-age development. In: Tasman A, Kay J, Lieberman JA *et al.* (eds.). *Psychiatry*, 3rd edn. Wiley: Oxford, 2008: 150–160.
6. Towbin KE, Showalter JE. Adolescent development. In: Tasman A, Kay J, Lieberman JA *et al.* (eds.). *Psychiatry*, 3rd edn. Wiley: Oxford, 2008: 161–180.
7. Vaillant G. *Adaptation to Life*. Harvard University Press: Cambridge, 1977.

Recommended Reading: Part Four

Chapter 13

1. Fonagy P, Gergely G, Jurist E *et al. Affect Regulation, Mentalization and the Development of the Self*. Other Press: New York, 2002.
2. Frankl V. *Man's Search for Meaning*. Beacon Press: Boston, 1959.
3. Herman J. *Trauma and Recovery*. Basic Books: New York, 1992.
4. Kellerman N. *Holocaust Trauma: Psychological Effects and Treatment*. iUniverse, Inc.: Bloomington, 2009.
5. Shengold L. *Soul Murder: The Effects of Childhood Abuse and Deprivation*. Fawcett Columbine: New York, 1989.
6. Terr LD. Childhood traumas: An outline and overview. *American Journal of Psychiatry* 1991; **148**: 10–20.
7. van der Kolk B. The body keeps the score: Memory & the evolving psychobiology of post traumatic stress. *Harvard Review of Psychiatry* 1994; **1** (5): 253–265.
8. Yovell Y. From hysteria to posttraumatic stress disorder: Psychoanalysis and the neurobiology of traumatic memories. *Neuropsychoanalysis* 2000; **2**: 171–181.

Chapter 14

1. Andrews G, Pine DS, Hobbs MJ *et al.* Neurodevelopmental disorders: Cluster 2 of the proposed meta-structure for DSM-V and ICD-11. *Psychological Medicine* 2009; **39** (12): 2013–2023.
2. Bernard S. Mental health and behavioural problems in children and adolescents with learning disabilties. *Psychiatry* 2009; **8**: 387–390.
3. Buitelaar J, Kan C, Asherson P. *ADHD in Adults: Characterization, Diagnosis, and Treatment*. Cambridge University Press: Cambridge, 2011.

4. Costello EJ, Mustillo S, Erkanli A *et al.* Prevalence and development of psychiatric disorders in childhood and adolescence. *Archives of General Psychiatry* 2003; **60**: 837–844.
5. Kim-Cohen J, Caspi A, Moffitt TE *et al.* Prior juvenile diagnoses in adults with mental disorder: Developmental follow-back of a prospective-longitudinal cohort. *Archives of General Psychiatry* 2003; **60** (7): 709–717.
6. Sachdev P, Andrews G, Hobbs MJ *et al.* Neurocognitive disorders: Cluster 1 of the proposed meta-structure for DSM-V and ICD-11. *Psychological Medicine* 2009; **39** (12): 2001–2012.
7. Soloman M, Hessl D, Chiu S *et al.* Towards a neurodevelopmental model of clinical case formulation. *Psychiatric Clinics of North America* 2009; **32** (1): 199–211.

Chapter 15

1. Brenner C. *An Elementary Textbook of Psychoanalysis (Revised and Expanded Edition)*. Anchor Books: New York, 1974.
2. Freud A. *The Ego and the Mechanisms of Defense*. Hogarth Press: London, 1937.
3. Gottlieb RM. Classical psychoanalysis: Past and present. In: *Textbook of Psychoanalysis*, 2nd edn. American Psychiatric Publishing, Inc: Washington, DC, 2012.
4. Mitchell SA, Black MJ. *Freud and Beyond*. Basic Books: New York, 1995.

Chapter 16

1. Fairburn WRD. *An Object-Relations Theory of Personality*. Basic Books: New York, 1954.
2. Fonagy P, Target M. *Psychoanalytic Theories: Perspectives from Developmental Psychology*. Brunner-Routledge: New York, 2003.
3. Greenberg J, Mitchell S. *Object Relations in Psychoanalytic Theory*. Harvard University Press: Boston, 1983.
4. Kernberg OF. *Object Relations Theory and Clinical Psychoanalysis*. Aronson: New York, 1976.
5. Kernberg OF. An ego-psychology object relations approach to the transference. *Psychoanalytic Quarterly* 1987; **57**: 481–504.
6. Klein M. *Contributions to Psychoanalysis, 1921-1945*. Hogarth Press: London, 1948.
7. Sullivan HS. *The Interpersonal Theory of Psychiatry*. W.W. Norton & Co.: New York, 1953.
8. Winnicott DW. *Collected Papers*. Basic Books: New York, 1958.

Chapter 17

1. Fonagy P, Target M. *Psychoanalytic Theories: Perspectives from Developmental Psychology*. Brunner-Routledge: New York, 2003.
2. Kohut H. *The Analysis of the Self*. The University of Chicago Press: Chicago, 1971.
3. Kohut H. *The Restoration of the Self*. The University of Chicago Press: Chicago, 1977.
4. Kohut H. The two analyses of Mr. Z. *International Journal of Psychoanalysis* 1979; **60**: 3–27.
5. Kohut H, Wolf ES. The disorders of the self and their treatment: An outline. *International Journal of Psychoanalysis* 1978; **59**: 413–425.
6. Kohut H, Goldberg A (eds.). *How Does Analysis Cure?* The University of Chicago Press: Chicago, 1984.
7. Mitchell S, Black M. *Freud and Beyond: A History of Modern Psychoanalytic Thought*. Basic Books: New York, 1995.
8. Stolorow RD. Toward a functional definition of narcissism. *International Journal of Psychoanalysis* 1975; **56**: 179–185.

Chapter 18

1. Bowlby J. The nature of the child's tie to his mother. *International Journal of Psychoanalysis* 1958; **39**: 350–373.
2. Fonagy P. *Attachment Theory and Psychoanalysis*. Other Press: New York, 2001.
3. Slade A. The development and organization of attachment: Implications for psychoanalysis. *Journal of the American Psychoanalytic Association* 2000; **48**: 1147–1174.
4. Stern DN. *The Interpersonal World of the Infant*. Basic Books: New York, 1985.

Recommended Reading: Part Five

Chapter 19

1. MacKinnon RA, Michels R, Buckley PJ. *The Psychiatric Interview in Clinical Practice*. American Psychiatric Publishing, Inc.: Washington, DC, 2006.
2. Schwartz HJ, Bleiberg E, Weissman SH. *Psychodynamic Concepts in General Psychiatry*. American Psychiatric Publishing, Inc.: Washington, DC, 1995.

Chapter 20

1. Busch FN, Auchincloss EL. The psychology of prescribing and taking medication. In: Schwartz H, Bleiberg E, Weissman S (eds.). *Psychodynamic Concepts in General Psychiatry*. American Psychiatric Publishing, Inc.: Arlington, 1995: 401–416.
2. Busch FN, Sandberg LS. *Psychotherapy and Medication: The Challenge of Integration*. Analytic Press: New York, 2007.
3. Roose SP, Cabaniss DL, Rutherford BR. Combining psychoanalysis and psychopharmacology: Theory and technique. In: Gabbard GO, Litowitz BE, Williams P (eds.). *Textbook of Psychoanalysis*, 2nd edn. American Psychiatric Publishing, Inc.: Washington, DC, 2012: 319–332.

Chapter 22

1. Summers RF, Barber JP. *Psychodynamic Therapy: A Guide to Evidence-Based Practice*. Guilford Press: New York, 2010.
2. Bateman A, Brown D, Pedder J. *Introduction to Psychotherapy: An Outline of Psychodynamic Principles and Practice*, 4th edn. Tavistock, Routledge: New York, 2010.
3. Perry SW, Cooper A, Michels R. The psychodynamic formulation: Its purpose, structure and clinical applications. *American Journal of Psychiatry* 1987; **144**: 543–550.

Index

abuse, childhood 148
accidental factors 5
acute care settings, psychodynamic
    formulation in 215–21
adapting 41–51
    definition of 41
    describing 50
    impact of trauma on 147
    variables for describing 42
adolescence 115–17
    adult problems and patterns that
        suggest an origin in 116–17
adulthood 118–19
affective attunement 96
affective regulation (see managing
    emotions)
Ainsworth, Mary 92
alcohol, affect on development 84
antisocial tendencies 115
anxiety disorders 82, 84–5, 107, 153,
    155
attachment 14, 191–9
    insecure attachment in adults
        192–4
    insecure attachment in children 93
    intergenerational transmission of
        194
    secure attachment 35, 92–3
attachment styles 192
attachment theory 192
attention deficit hyperactivity disorder
    (ADHD) 82, 84, 115, 153

attitude toward illness 225
attitude toward medication 225
autism 82, 84–5, 153

Balint, Michael 174
bipolar disorder 153
Bowlby, John 94, 174

causative links 6
cerebral palsy 85
chronology 77
cigarette smoking, affect on
    development 84
cognition 52–60
    definition of 52
    describing 59
    variables for describing 53
cognitive and emotional difficulties
    152–62
    impact of parental response and
        early treatment on 156
    in adolescence 116, 155
    in adulthood 156
    in childhood 153
cognitive development in later
    childhood 114
commitment, difficulties
    with 167
competition 27
competitive anxiety 166
conduct disorder 155

Psychodynamic Formulation, First Edition. Deborah L. Cabaniss, Sabrina Cherry, Carolyn J. Douglas,
Ruth L. Graver, and Anna R. Schwartz.
© 2013 John Wiley & Sons, Ltd. Published 2013 by John Wiley & Sons, Ltd.

conflict and defense   163–72
  compromise   163
  definition of   163
  unconscious conflict and   164
cultural factors in development   115,
  118

defenses   42–6
  definition of   164
  flexibility of   43–6
  in middle childhood   103
  more and less adaptive defenses
    43, 165–6
  relationship to thoughts and feelings
    46
  table of   44–5
deferred action   105
denial   43
depression   84, 154
Descartes, Rene   52
describing problems and patterns   13,
  17–21
devaluation   43
Diagnostic and Statistical Manual of
  Mental Disorders (DSM)   19
dimensions of function   20
Disorders of Extreme Stress Not
  Otherwise Specified (DESNOS)
  144
dyadic relationship   91, 101
  definition of   91

earliest years, the   90–100
  adult problems and patterns that
    suggest origins in   97
eating disorders   155
egg donation   89
ego   164
ego function   114
ego psychology   164
emergency room, psychiatric   214,
  217
empathic failure   188
empathic responsiveness   96
empathy   28, 94
  problems with   186, 195
enuresis/encopresis   154

envy   26, 186
Erikson, Erik   113

Fairbairn, W.R.D.   174
fantasies
  about the self   25
  unconscious   117
fear of competition   109
fetal alcohol syndrome   84
formulation, definition of   3
foundation, internal   91
Freud, Sigmund   5, 19
  structural model   164
  topographical model   164

general cognitive ability   53
  decision making and problem
    solving   54–5
  describing   59
  judgment   56
  mentalization (see mentalization)
  self-reflection   55
  table of   53
genetics   5, 81–3
  adult problems that suggest a
    genetic origin   86–7
  genes and environment
    interrelationships   5–6
  genetic endowment   81
"good enough" parenting   91
grandiosity   27, 183
Guntrip, Harry   174

Hippocrates   19
histories
  of present illness   76
  past psychiatric   76

id   164
idealization   43
identification   103, 174
identity   24, 115–16
  sexual   116
impulse control   47–8
  impact of trauma on   146
inhibitions, sexual   108
insight   242

intimacy   32, 35–6, 117
  difficulties with   167

jealousy   26

Kagan, Jerome   83
Kohut, Heinz   183

later childhood   113–22
  adult problems and patterns that
      suggest origins in   115
learning disorders   153
life cycle   78, 113, 121
life narrative, creating   10, 241–2
linking problems and patterns to
      history   135–41
  language of   139
  linking to attachment styles   195–7
  linking to conflict and defense
      168–9
  linking to development of the self
      184–8
  linking to the impact of early
      cognitive and emotional
      difficulties   157–9
  linking to relationships with others
      176–9
  linking to trauma   145–9
Locke, John   5
low birth weight, affect on
      development   85

managing emotions   46, 96
  development of ability to   194
  impact of trauma on   146
  problems with   195
masochism   27
masturbation   116
"med check"   222
mentalization   34, 56, 94
middle childhood   101–12
  adult problems and patterns that
      suggest origins in   108–9
mirroring   183
mood disorders   82, 154
moral development   107
mutuality in relationships   36

narcissistic injury   25
nature and nurture   76

object constancy   94
  impact of trauma on   148
object permanence   94
object relations theory   173
oedipus complex   102
oedipal fantasies   105
oedipal phase   103
oedipal victor   104
organizing ideas about development
      138–9

person, the   19–20
post-traumatic stress disorder (PTSD)
      144
prematurity, affect on development
      85
prenatal development   83
  maternal habits and   84
  maternal physical and emotional
      health and   84
primary caregiver   91
  connecting to   91
  definition of   91
problem, the   18–19
psychodynamic frame of reference   4
psychodynamic psychotherapy,
      long-term   230–237
psychological mindedness   55
psychopharmacologic treatment,
      psychodynamic formulations in
      222–9

reality testing   55
relationships with others   32–40, 106,
      173–81
  definition of   32
  describing   39
  impact of trauma on   146–7
  variables for describing   32–3
repression   167
resilience   86
reviewing the developmental history
      13
revising formulations   230–237

sample formulations
    in acute care settings   217
    in long-term psychodynamic
        psychotherapy   233, 236
    in psychopharmacologic treatment
        227–9
    linking to attachment style   196–7
    linking to cognitive and emotional
        difficulties   159–161
    linking to conflict/defense   168–169
    linking to development of the self
        187–8
    linking to relationships with others
        177–9
    linking to trauma   148–9
schizophrenia   84
security   32, 35
self   23–31
    definition of   23
    describing   30
    development of   182–90
    variables for describing   24
self-esteem   25, 95
    development of   182
    fragility   26
    regulation of   25, 105, 185–6
self-esteem threat   25
    responses to   26–9
self-experience   23, 95
    impact of trauma on   145
self-perception   24
self psychology   183
selfobject   183
sense of self and other   34
sensory regulation   48
separation anxiety disorder   153
setting goals in psychotherapy   9
sharing formulations with patients
        10–11, 238–43
siblings   106
somatization   167
split treatment   223
splitting   43, 165
stimulation
    external   42
    internal   41

strange situation   92
strengths and difficulties   20
sublimation   165
substance abuse   155
    in adolescence   116
super-ego   107, 164
supervisors   251–2
supporting   170–171

tactile stimulation, need for early in life
        91
temperament   82
    easy, difficulty and slow to warm up
        temperaments   83
    impulsive aggressivity   83
    inhibited temperament   83
    sensation seeking   83
    uninhibited temperament   83
templates, for relationships   174
termination   242
therapeutic strategy   9
tics, motor and verbal   154
transference   179
trauma   14, 76–7, 143–51
    definition of   143
    impact on development   144
treatment recommendations   9,
        240–241
triadic relationship   102
trust   32–3, 92

uncovering   170

Valliant, George   119

Wilson, E.O.   5
Winnicott, Donald   91, 174
work and play   61–8
    definitions of   61–2
    describing   66–7
    variables for describing   63–5

young adulthood   117–18
    adult problems and patterns that
        suggest origins in   118